AF820762

Official Journal of the 'Mediterranean League against Thromboembolic Diseases'

Hæmostasis

International Journal on Haemostasis and Thrombosis Research

Managing Editor

H.C. Hemker, Maastricht

Associate Editors

S. Levy-Toledano, Paris
T. Lindhout, Maastricht
J. Rosing, Maastricht

Editorial Secretary

T. Camphuisen-Engel, Maastricht

Editorial Committee

G. Agnelli, Perugia
M. Aiach, Paris
R. Altman, Buenos Aires
R. Apitz-Castro, Caracas
J. Aznar, Valencia
J.J. Badimon, New York, N.Y.
G. Baele, Gent
S. Béguin, Maastricht
B. Boneu, Toulouse
N.B. de Bosch, Caracas
H.K. Breddin, Frankfurt
M.R. Buchanan, Hamilton, Ont.
H.R. Büller, Amsterdam
S. Coccheri, Bologna
B.S. Coller, New York, N.Y.
J. Conard, Paris
F. DeClerck, Beerse
A. Eldor, Tel-Aviv
E. Gray, Hertfordshire
D. Green, Chicago, Ill.
U. Hedner, Gentofte
D.L. Heene, Mannheim
J. Jesty, Stony Brook, N.Y.
B. Jørgensen, Aalborg
I. Juhan-Vague, Marseille
B. Kemkes-Matthes, Giessen
W. Kisiel, Albuquerque, N. Mex.
D. Lane, London
A.K. Lindahl, Uppsala
F. Lupu, London
Ma Xi, Xian
J. Monasterio-Aspiri, Barcelona
M. Mosesson, Milwaukee, Wisc.
H. Pannekoek, Amsterdam
G. Potron, Reims
K.T. Preissner, Giessen
M.H. Prins, Amsterdam
J.H. Rand, New York, N.Y.
L.V.M. Rao, Tyler, Tex.
P.H. Reitsma, Amsterdam
J.F. Schved, Montpellier
M.F. Scully, London
D.A. Triplett, Muncie, Ind.
A. Uzan, Vitry-sur-Seine
J.M. Walenga, Maywood, Ill.
J. Yamamoto, Kobe
L. Yukelson, Tashkent

KARGER

Printed in Switzerland on acid-free paper by Reinhardt Druck, Basel

Appears bimonthly: 1 volume per year (6 issues)

Guidelines for Authors

Hæmostasis

Submission

Only original papers written in English that communicate novel findings in the field of haemostasis and thrombosis are considered. Both contributions to the basic understanding of these processes and reports on clinical management of disorders in this field are acceptable. Manuscripts can be sent either to the managing editor or to one of the editors as listed in each issue of Haemostasis.
Manuscripts should be submitted in triplicate (with three sets of illustrations of which one is an original), typewritten double-spaced on one side of the paper, with a wide margin.

Conditions

All manuscripts are subject to editorial review. A manuscript is to be considered rejected when an author does not return a revised manuscript within 3 months of receiving the suggestions for revision, unless the author explains further delay. Manuscripts are received with the explicit understanding that they are not under simultaneous consideration by any other publication. Submission of an article for publication implies the transfer of the copyright from the author to the publisher upon acceptance. Accepted papers become the permanent property of 'Haemostasis' and may not be reproduced by any means, in whole or in part, without the written consent of both the author and the publisher. It is the author's responsibility to obtain permission to reproduce illustrations, tables, etc. from other publications.

Arrangement

Title page: The first page of each paper should indicate the title (main title underlined), the authors' names, and the institute where the work was conducted. A short title for use as running head as well as the full address of the author to whom correspondence should be sent are also required.

Full address: The exact postal address complete with postal code must be given at the bottom of the title page. Please also supply phone and fax numbers, as well as your e-mail address.

Key words: For indexing purposes, a list of 3–10 key words in English is essential.

Abstract: Each paper needs an abstract of up to 10 lines.

Small type: Paragraphs which can or must be set in smaller type (case histories, test methods, etc.) should be indicated with a 'p' (petit) in the margin on the left-hand side.

Footnotes: Avoid footnotes. When essential, they are numbered consecutively and typed at the foot of the appropriate page.

Tables and illustrations: Tables and illustrations (both numbered in Arabic numerals) should be prepared on separate sheets. Tables require a heading and figures a legend, also prepared on a separate sheet. For the reproduction of illustrations, only good drawings and original photographs can be accepted; negatives or photocopies cannot be used. Due to technical reasons, figures with a screen background should not be submitted. When possible, group several illustrations on one block for reproduction (max. size 144 × 196 mm) or provide crop marks. On the back of each illustration, indicate its number, the author's name, and 'top' with a soft pencil.

Color illustrations: Up to 6 color illustrations per page can be integrated with the text at the reduced price of CHF 660.– / USD 545.00 per page. Color illustrations are reproduced at the author's expense.

References: In the text identify references by Arabic numerals [in square brackets]. Material submitted for publication but not yet accepted should be noted as 'unpublished data' and not be included in the reference list. The list of references should include only those publications which are cited in the text. Do not alphabetize; number references in the order in which they are first mentioned in the text. The surnames of the authors followed by initials should be given. There should be no punctuation other than a comma to separate the authors. Cite all authors, 'et al' is not sufficient. Abbreviate journal names according to the Index Medicus system. (Also see International Committee of Medical Journal Editors: Uniform requirements for manuscripts submitted to biomedical journals. N Engl J Med 1997;336:309–315.)

(a) Papers published in periodicals: Sun J, Koto H, Chung KF: Interaction of ozone and allergen challenges on bronchial responsiveness and inflammation in sensitised guinea pigs. Int Arch Allergy Immunol 1997;112:191–195.

(b) Monographs: Matthews DE, Farewell VT: Using and Understanding Medical Statistics, ed 3, revised. Basel, Karger, 1996.

(c) Edited books: Parren PWHI, Burton DR: Antibodies against HIV-1 from phage display libraries: Mapping of an immune response and progress towards antiviral immunotherapy; in Capra JD (ed): Antibody Engineering. Chem Immunol. Basel, Karger, 1997, vol 65, pp 18–56.

Page charges

There is no page charge for papers of 6 or fewer printed pages (including tables, illustrations and references). Each additional complete or partial page is charged to the author at CHF 275.– / USD 196.00. The allotted size of a paper is equal to approx. 12 manuscript pages (including tables, illustrations and references).

Galley proofs

Unless indicated otherwise, galley proofs are sent to the first-named author and should be returned with the least possible delay. Alterations made in galley proofs, other than the correction of printer's errors, are charged to the author. No page proofs are supplied.

Reprints

Order forms and a price list are sent with the galley proofs. Orders submitted after the issue is printed are subject to considerably higher prices.

KARGER

© 1999 S. Karger AG, Basel

Fax +41 61 306 12 34
E-Mail karger@karger.ch
www.karger.com

The Guidelines for Authors are available at:
www.karger.com/journals/hae/hae_gl.htm

Hæmostasis

General Information

Publication data: 'Haemostasis' is published 6 times a year. Volume 28 with 6 issues appears in 1998.

Subscription rates: Subscriptions run for a full calendar year. Prices are given per volume.

Personal subscription:
Subscription + postage and handling
CHF 258.– + CHF 23.50 Europe
CHF 258.– + CHF 35.50 Overseas
USD 201.00 + USD 23.50
(Must be in the name of, billed to, and paid by an individual. Order must be marked 'personal subscription'.)

Institutional subscription:
Subscription + postage and handling
CHF 516.– + CHF 29.40 Europe
CHF 516.– + CHF 44.40 Overseas
USD 402.00 + USD 29.40

Airmail postage: CHF 36.–, USD 30.00.
(Extra per volume.)

Discount subscription prices:
Gesellschaft für Thrombose- und Haemostase-Forschung;
International Society of Haematology.

Microforms: Please direct all enquiries and orders to: University Microfilms Inc.
300 North Zeeb Road, P.O. Box 1346
Ann Arbor, MI 48106-1346 (USA)

Subscription orders: Orders can be placed at agencies, bookstores, directly with the
Publisher S. Karger AG, P.O. Box,
CH–4009 Basel (Switzerland)
or with any of the following distributors:

Deutschland: S. Karger GmbH, Postfach
D–79095 Freiburg

France: Librairie Luginbühl
36, bd de Latour-Maubourg
F–75007 Paris

Great Britain, Ireland: S. Karger Publishers
58 Grove Hill Road
Tunbridge Wells, Kent TN1 1SP

USA: S. Karger Publishers, Inc.
26 West Avon Road, P.O. Box 529
Farmington, CT 06085

India, Bangladesh, Sri Lanka:
S. Karger India Subscription Agency
B–5/132 Safdarjung Enclave
New Delhi-110029

Japan: Katakura Libri, Inc.
2F, Marushima Bldg,
4-6-17, Yushima,Bunkyo-ku,
Tokyo 113-0034

Change of address: Both old and new address should be sent to the subscription source.

Single issues and back volumes: Information can be obtained through the Publisher.

Advertising: Correspondence and rate requests should be addressed to the Publisher.

Bibliographic indices: This journal is regularly listed in bibliographic services, including *Current Contents®*.

Copying: This journal has been registered with the Copyright Clearance Center (CCC), as indicated by the code appearing on the first page of each article.
For readers in the US, this code signals consent for copying of articles for personal or internal use, or for the personal or internal use of specific clients, provided that the stated fee is paid per copy directly to
Copyright Clearance Center Inc.
222 Rosewood Drive
Danvers, MA 01923 (USA).
A copy of the first page of the article must accompany payment. Consent does not extend to copying for general distribution, for promotion, for creating new works, or for resale. In these cases, specific written permission must be obtained from the copyright owner,
S. Karger AG, P.O. Box,
CH–4009 Basel (Switzerland).

Hæmostasis

List of Editors

Dr. G. Agnelli
Istituto di Medicina Interna e Vascolare
Università di Perugia
Via Enrico dal Pozzo
I–06100 Perugia (Italy)

Prof. M. Aiach
Hôpital Broussais
Laboratoire d'Hémostase
96, rue Didot
F–75674 Paris Cedex 14 (France)

Dr. R. Altman
Centro de Estudios Médicos y Bioquímicos (CEMEBI)
Viamonte 2008
1056 Buenos Aires (Argentina)

Prof. R. Apitz-Castro
Instituto Venezolano de Investigaciones Cientificas (IVIC)
Caracas 1020 A (Venezuela)

Dr. J. Aznar
Department of Clinical Pathology
'La Fe' University Hospital
Avda Campanar, 21
E–46009 Valencia (Spain)

Dr. J.J. Badimon
Associate Professor of Medicine
The Cardiovascular Institute (Box 1030)
One Gustave L. Levy Place
New York, NY 10029 (USA)

Prof. G. Baele
Coagulation Laboratory
University Hospital
De Pintelaan 185
B–9000 Gent (Belgium)

Dr. S. Béguin
Universiteit Maastricht
Department of Biochemistry
Faculty of Medicine II, Level 4
P.O. Box 616
NL–6200 MD Maastricht (The Netherlands)

Prof. B. Boneu
Laboratoire d'Hématologie
Hôpital de Rangueil
F–31054 Toulouse Cedex (France)

Prof. N.B. de Bosch
Departamento de Investigaciones y Centro Nacional de Hemofilia
Banco Municipal de Sangre
Apartado Postal 6782
Caracas 1010 (Venezuela)

Prof. Dr. H.K. Breddin
Center of Internal Medicine
J.W. Goethe University
Division of Angiology
Theodor-Stern-Kai 7
D–60596 Frankfurt am Main (Germany)

Dr. M.R. Buchanan
Professor of Pathology
McMaster University
293 Wellington St. North, Suite 132
Hamilton, Ont. L8L 8E7 (Canada)

Dr. H.R. Büller
Center for Hemostasis, Thrombosis, Atherosclerosis and Inflammation Research
Academic Medical Center
Meibergdreef 9
NL–1105 AZ Amsterdam (The Netherlands)

Mrs. T. Camphuisen-Engel (Editorial Secretary)
Universiteit Maastricht
Department of Biochemistry
Faculty of Medicine II, Level 4
PO Box 616
NL–6200 MD Maastricht (The Netherlands)

KARGER

Fax+ 41 61 306 12 34
E-Mail karger@karger.ch
www.karger.com

© 1999 S. Karger AG, Basel

The Journal Home Page is available at:
www.karger.com/journals/hae

List of Editors (continued)

Hæmostasis

Prof. S. Coccheri
Professor of Cardiovascular Diseases
Director of the Division of Angiology and Blood Coagulation
University of Bologna
Via Massarenti 9
I–40138 Bologna (Italy)

Dr. B.S. Coller
Department of Medicine
The Mount Sinai Medical Center
One Gustave L. Levy Place
Box 1118
New York, NY 10029-6574 (USA)

Dr. J. Conard
Hôtel-Dieu de Paris
Lab Central d'Hématologie
1, place du Parvis Notre-Dame
F–75181 Paris Cedex 04 (France)

Prof. F. De Clerck
Head Department Cardiovascular Pharmacology
Janssen Research Foundation
Turnhoutseweg 30
B–2340 Beerse (Belgium)

Dr. A. Eldor
Prof. of Medicine
Institute of Hematology
Tel-Aviv Souraski
Medical Center
6 Weizman Street
Tel-Aviv 64239 (Israel)

Dr. E. Gray
Division of Haematology
National Institute for Biological Standards and Control (NIBSC)
Blanche Lane, South Mimms
Potters Bar
Hertfordshire EN6 3QG (UK)

Prof. D. Green
Northwestern University Medical School
Rehabilitation Institute of Chicago
345 E. Superior St. Room 1407
Chicago, IL 60611 (USA)

Prof. U. Hedner
Research Biopharmaceuticals Division
Novo Nordisk A/S
Niels Steensens Vej 1
DK–2820 Gentofte (Denmark)

Prof. D.L. Heene
Professor of Medicine
I. Department of Medicine
Faculty of Clinical Medicine
University of Heidelberg
Theodor-Kutzer-Ufer
D–68167 Mannheim (Germany)

Prof. H.C. Hemker (Managing Editor)
Universiteit Maastricht
Department of Biochemistry
Faculty of Medicine II, Level 4
P.O. Box 616
NL–6200 MD Maastricht (The Netherlands)

Prof. J. Jesty
Division of Hematology
Health Sciences Center
State University of New York
Stony Brook, NY 11794-8151 (USA)

Dr. B. Jørgensen
Department of Clinical Chemistry
Aalborg Hospital, section South
DK–9100 Aalborg (Denmark)

Dr. I. Juhan-Vague
Laboratory of Hematology
Internal Medicine Department
CHU Timone
Bd Jean-Moulin
F–13385 Marseille Cedex 5 (France)

Dr. B. Kemkes-Matthes
Zentrum Innere Medizin
Klinikstrasse 36
D–35385 Giessen (Germany)

Dr. W. Kisiel
Department of Pathology
University of New Mexico
School of Medicine
Albuquerque, NM 87131 (USA)

Dr. D. Lane
Charing Cross Hospital
Fulham Palace Road
London W68 RF (UK)

Dr. S. Levy-Toledano (Associate Editor)
INSERM Unite 150
Hôpital Lariboisière
6, rue Guy-Patin
F–75010 Paris (France)

Dr. A.K. Lindahl
Biomedical Center
Box 575
S–751 23 Uppsala (Sweden)

Dr. F. Lupu
Vascular Biology Laboratory
Thrombosis Research Institute
Emmanuel Kaye Building
Manresa Road, Chelsea
London SW3 6LR (UK)

Dr. Ma Xi
Research Unit for Experimental Hematology
Xian Medical University
205 Scarlet Bird Ave.
Xian 710061 (P.R. China)

Prof. J. Monasterio-Aspiri
Head Unit de Recerça d'Hemostasia
Ciutat Sanitaria Vall d'Hebro
Po Vall d'Hebro s/n
E–8034 Barcelona (Spain)

Prof. Michael W. Mosesson
Sinai Samaritan Medical Center
950 North 12th Street
Milwaukee, WI 53233 (USA)

Prof. H. Pannekoek
University of Amsterdam
Academic Medical Center
Department of Biochemistry
Meibergdreef 15
NL–1105 AZ Amsterdam (The Netherlands)

Prof. G. Potron
Laboratoire d'Hématologie
Centre Hospitalier Universitaire Robert-Debré
F–51092 Reims Cedex (France)

Prof. K.T. Preissner
Institut für Biochemie
Fachbereich Humanmedizin
Justus-Liebig-Universität
Friedrichstrasse 24
D–35392 Giessen (Germany)

Dr. M.H. Prins
Academic Medical Center
University of Amsterdam
Department of Clinical Epidemiology & Biostatistics
Meibergdreef 9
NL–1105 AZ Amsterdam (The Netherlands)

Dr. J.H. Rand
Prof. of Medicine/Hematology
Director, Coagulation Laboratory
The Mount Sinai Medical Center
One Gustave L. Levy Place
New York, NY 10029-6574 (USA)

Dr. L. Vijaya Mohan Rao
University of Texas Health Center at Tyler
Department of Biochemistry
P.O. Box 2003
Tyler, TX 75710 (USA)

Dr. P.H. Reitsma
Laboratory of Experimental Internal Medicine
Academic Medical Center, Room G2-132
Meibergdreef 9
NL–1105 AZ Amsterdam (The Netherlands)

Prof. J.F. Schved
Laboratoire d'Hématologie
Centre Hôpitalier Universitaire de Montpellier
F–34295 Montpellier Cedex 5 (France)

Dr. M.F. Scully
Thrombosis Research Institute
Emmanuel Kaye Building
Manresa Road, Chelsea
London SW3 6LR (UK)

Dr. D.A. Triplett
Vice President/Director, Medical Education
Ball Memorial Hospital
2401 University Avenue
Muncie, IN 47303 (USA)

Dr. A. Uzan
RPR Thrombosis Research
Centre de Recherches de Vitry
13, quai Jules-Guesdes
BP 14
F–94403 Vitry-sur-Seine (France)

Dr. J.M. Walenga
Cardiovascular Institute
Loyola University Medical Center
2160 S. First Ave.
Maywood, IL 60153 (USA)

Prof. J. Yamamoto
Laboratory of Physiology
Faculty of Nutrition
Kobe-Gakuin University
Nishi-ku, Kobe 651-21 (Japan)

Prof. L. Yukelson
Academy of Sciences of Uzbek Soviet Socialistic Republic
Institute of Biochemistry
Prospect M.G. Gorky 55
7001143 Tashkent (Uzbekistan)

KARGER

© 1999 S. Karger AG, Basel

Fax+ 41 61 306 12 34
E-Mail karger@karger.ch
www.karger.com

The Journal Home Page is available at:
www.karger.com/journals/hae

Hæmostasis

Thromboembolism: New Achievements and Challenges

Proceedings of the 6th International Symposium on Thromboembolic Diseases
Lisbon, June 4–5, 1999

Editors
Sylvia Haas, Munich
Mark Levine, Hamilton, Ont.
Meyer-Michel Samama, Paris

KARGER

Basel · Freiburg · Paris · London · New York ·
New Delhi · Bangkok · Singapore · Tokyo · Sydney

S. Karger
Medical and Scientific Publishers
Basel · Freiburg · Paris · London
New York · New Delhi · Bangkok
Singapore · Tokyo · Sydney

Drug Dosage
The authors and the publisher have exerted every effort to ensure that drug selection and dosage set forth in this text are in accord with current recommendations and practice at the time of publication. However, in view of ongoing research, changes in government regulations, and the constant flow of information relating to drug therapy and drug reactions, the reader is urged to check the package insert for each drug for any change in indications and dosage and for added warnings and precautions. This is particularly important when the recommended agent is a new and/or infrequently employed drug.

All rights reserved.
No part of this publication may be translated into other languages, reproduced or utilized in any form or by any means, electronic or mechanical, including photocopying, recording, microcopying, or by any information storage and retrieval system, without permission in writing from the publisher or, in the case of photocopying, direct payment of a specified fee to the Copyright Clearance Center (see 'General Information').

© Copyright 1999 by S. Karger AG,
P.O. Box, CH–4009 Basel (Switzerland)
Printed in Switzerland on acid-free paper by Reinhardt Druck, Basel
ISBN 3–8055–7041–4

KARGER

Fax+ 41 61 306 12 34
E-Mail karger@karger.ch
www.karger.com

Hæmostasis

Contents Vol. 29, Suppl. 1, 1999

KARGER

Fax+41 61 306 12 34
E-Mail karger@karger.ch
www.karger.com

© 1999 S. Karger AG, Basel

Access to full text and tables of contents, including tentative ones for forthcoming issues:
www.karger.com/journals/hae/hae_bk.htm

Preface

Sylvia Haas[a] Mark Levine[b] Meyer-Michel Samama[c]

[a] Institut für Experimentelle Onkologie und Therapieforschung, Technical University, Munich, Germany, [b] Hamilton Regional Cancer Centre, Hamilton, Ont., Canada, [c] Hôpital Hôtel-Dieu, Paris, France

In the past decade we have witnessed many exciting advances in the diagnosis and treatment of patients with thromboembolic disease. These advances have occurred because of an improved understanding of the molecular biology of haemostasis and thrombosis, the development of new antithrombotic agents, and the fact that rigorous clinical trials evaluating both new and old agents have been conducted.

Some years ago, Professor V.V. Kakkar of the Thrombosis Research Institute, London, UK, initiated a series of international meetings in order to discuss the state of the art of antithrombotic therapy. In June 1999, the sixth such symposium was held in Lisbon, Portugal. The International Symposium on Thromboembolism: New Achievements and Challenges was held as a forum where recent data were considered, controversies were discussed and areas for future research were identified by clinicians and researchers from all over the world.

In choosing the topics for the plenary sessions and workshops we tried to identify themes relevant both to the routine management of patients with thromboembolic disease (e.g. Frontiers in diagnosis, prophylaxis and treatment of VTE) and to the non-thrombotic areas which could have major relevance in the future (e.g. Non-antithrombotic properties of heparins: Future use potential?). Attendees were also encouraged to submit abstracts for poster presentations.

The Editors would like to express their sincere thanks to the authors who have contributed to the proceedings. We also greatly appreciate the enthusiasm exhibited by the attendees at the symposium. Great thanks should also be given to Dr. Rolf Gunnarsson and Ms Annika Nyman from Pharmacia & Upjohn for the effective organization of the symposium. Thanks also to REMEDICA Communications for their help in producing this permanent record of the meeting.

KARGER

Fax + 41 61 306 12 34
E-Mail karger@karger.ch
www.karger.com

© 1999 S. Karger AG, Basel

Accessible online at:
www.karger.com/journals/hae

Main Paper

Hæmostasis

Haemostasis 1999;29(suppl 1)1–9

Venous Thrombosis: Prevalence and Interaction of Risk Factors

F.R. Rosendaal

University Hospital Leiden, Leiden, The Netherlands

Key Words
Gene–gene interaction · Gene–environment interaction · Selection and interaction · Dynamic age-dependent model · Factor V Leiden · Factor VIII · Protein C deficiency

Abstract
The key to understanding why certain individuals develop deep vein thrombosis at varying times, despite similar risk factors being present, is the realization of the importance of gene–gene and gene–environment interactions between risk factors. The discovery of factor V Leiden and several other coagulation abnormalities, which are now known to be common in the general population, has revolutionized the way in which the aetiology of venous thrombosis is viewed. On the basis of current knowledge, time-dependent models taking account of various forms of interaction have been developed.

Copyright © 1999 S. Karger AG, Basel

Introduction

Thrombosis is a multicausal disease involving a variety of risk factors, many of which are common; it is now appreciated that the interaction of multiple risk factors over time determines the risk of thrombosis. It is often overlooked in comparisons between studies that one of the most important of these risk factors is age. In individuals aged less than 20 years, the incidence of venous thrombosis is 1 per 100,000 people; at middle age it is approximately 1 per 1,000, which is also the overall incidence; thereafter it increases steeply, and in old age approaches 1% per year.

Risk Factors

The risk factors for venous thrombosis are now generally classified as either genetic or acquired (table 1).

KARGER

Fax + 41 61 306 12 34
E-Mail karger@karger.ch
www.karger.com

© 1999 S. Karger AG, Basel
0301–0147/99/0297–0001$17.50/0

Accessible online at:
www.karger.com/journals/hae

Prof. F.R. Rosendaal
Department of Clinical Epidemiology
Blg 1. CO-P University Hospital Leiden
PO Box 9600
NL–2300 RC Leiden (The Netherlands)

Table 1. Main causes of venous thrombosis

Acquired	Genetic	Mixed
Surgery/trauma	Antithrombin deficiency	High levels of Factor VIII
Immobilization	Protein C deficiency	Hyperhomocysteinaemia
Lupus anticoagulant	Protein S deficiency	
Malignancy	Activated protein C resistance/Factor V Leiden	
Oestrogen		
Pregnancy/puerperium	Prothrombin 20210A	

From Rosendaal [33].

Egeberg [1], in 1965, was the first to establish a hereditary tendency to thrombosis when he recorded an inherited antithrombin deficiency within a family with thrombophilia. In the early 1980s, deficiencies of two natural anticoagulant proteins – protein C and protein S – were described in familial thrombophilia by Griffin et al. [2] and Schwartz et al. [3], respectively. Over the last 5 years, a variety of coagulation abnormalities predisposing to venous thrombosis have been identified. The first of these, described in 1993 by Dahlbäck et al. [4], was a previously unrecognized mechanism characterized by a poor anticoagulant response to activated protein C (APC), i.e. APC resistance. This was subsequently shown by Bertina et al. [5] in 1994 to be caused by a mutation in blood coagulation factor V, otherwise known as factor V Leiden. Heterozygous deficiency of the three major natural inhibitors of the procoagulant system – protein C, protein S and antithrombin – leads to excessive thrombin formation. Other abnormalities leading to gains in function and excesses in the procoagulant system include mutation of the prothrombin (factor II) gene, which is associated with raised plasma concentrations of prothrombin 20210A and an increased risk of thrombosis [6]. Raised concentrations of coagulation factor VIII, possibly caused by subtle changes in the regulation of gene activity [7], are also associated with an increased risk of thrombosis [8].

Variation due to Acquired Factors

Apart from genetic considerations, variations in the risk of venous thrombosis might also be explained by acquired factors or a combination of both acquired and genetic factors. Hyperhomocysteinaemia, which has been found to be associated with venous thrombosis in a number of studies [9–12], is a good example of abnormal plasma concentrations resulting from both genetic and acquired factors. It is also plausible that raised levels of factor VIII and prothrombin reflect a combination of genetic and acquired factors.

Prevalence and Risk Estimates

Even among patients with thrombosis, deficiencies of protein C, protein S and antithrombin (the classical deficiencies) are rare. Far more common in the general population are APC resistance, prothrombin 20210A, high concentrations of factor VIII, and hyperhomocysteinaemia. As shown in table 2 [6,

Table 2. Prevalence of risk factors for thrombosis

Risk factor	General population, %	Patients with thrombosis, %
Protein C deficiency	0.2–0.4	3
Protein S deficiency	Not known	1–2
Antithrombin deficiency	0.02	1
Factor V Leiden	5	20
Prothrombin 20210A	2	6
High concentration of factor VIII (>1,500 IU/l)	11	25
Hyperhomocysteinaemia (>18.5 μmol/l)	5	10

From Rosendaal [33].

13–18], 5% of the population have APC resistance as a result of factor V Leiden [17, 19]. Factor V Leiden is restricted to Caucasians, and regional differences are high. As shown in the table, factor V Leiden occurs in 20% of consecutive patients with venous thrombosis [17, 20] and increases the risk of thrombosis approximately eightfold among heterozygous carriers [17]. Prothrombin 20210A appears to be a relatively mild risk factor, increasing the risk of thrombosis by two- to threefold [6]. Again, this mutation has largely been reported in the white population [21]. Concentrations of factor VIII exceeding 1,500 IU/l have been detected in 11% of the general population and in 25% of thrombotic patients; such levels are associated with a sixfold increased risk of thrombosis as compared with concentrations below 1,000 IU/l [8].

The burden of deep vein thrombosis in society is largely explained by the latter four abnormalities, each of which is associated with a greater attributable risk than the three classical deficiencies combined. The discovery of factor V Leiden and an assessment of its prevalence in unselected patients with deep vein thrombosis (20%), patients with familial thrombosis (50%) and in the general population (5%) revolutionized the way in which the aetiology of thrombosis was viewed. Now that common risk factors had been identified, it became clear that there must be individuals having more than one risk factor. This realization led to attention being diverted to issues of selection and interaction.

Venous Thrombosis as a Multicausal Disorder

The demonstration that venous thrombosis is a multicausal disorder is most obvious in children. Although thrombosis is rare in children, in the event of it occurring, a variety of genetic and acquired risk factors are usually present simultaneously [22, 23]. The multicausality of thrombosis is also true in adults. In fact, for the development of thrombosis, multiple risk factors are a prerequisite.

Selection and Interaction

Among families with thrombophilia, thrombogenic abnormalities are far higher than in the unselected patient with thrombo-

Table 3. Age at first thrombosis by origin of patient

Risk factor	Age (years) at first thrombosis	
	patients from thrombophilic families (n = 78)	consecutive unselected patients (n = 105)
Protein C deficiency	31	47
Factor V Leiden	29	43
No defect found	34	46

From [33], with permission.

sis. In families with thrombophilia, the main coagulation inhibitors are deficient in 15% of individuals, prothrombin 20210A is evident in nearly 20%, and factor V Leiden occurs in 40–60%. Members of these families are also at higher risk for thrombosis than are other individuals with similar defects [5, 16, 24–29]. The most important determinant of an individual's thrombotic risk when comparing patients with the same defect appears to be the way in which they are identified or selected. Comparison between consecutive unselected patients and patients from families with thrombophilia indicates a lower mean age at first thrombosis for thrombophilic patients than for consecutive individuals with thrombosis, regardless of the underlying defect, as shown in table 3 [30].

The severity of thrombotic disease is defined here as the age at onset of the condition; the more severe the thrombotic tendency, the earlier the first thrombotic event occurs. Even in thrombophilic families with no identifiable defect, thrombosis occurs at an early age [31]. Why then does the same disorder with the same molecular basis manifest itself with greater severity in the thrombophilic population than in the unselected population? An explanation of this anomaly was found with the discovery of factor V Leiden, some 10 years after initial studies with thrombophilic patients had centred on the absence or presence of protein C deficiency. With the discovery of factor V Leiden, and further studies in familial thrombophilia, the role of gene–gene interaction and its influence on thrombosis-free survival became apparent.

Gene–Gene Interaction

It is now appreciated that although thrombosis is multicausal, in families with thrombophilia, it is also multigenic. That is, in each of the families studied, there are a variety of genetic defects. As shown in figure 1, members of families with thrombophilia were found in early studies to be at a high risk of thrombosis if they had protein C deficiency compared with relatives who did not have the deficiency [28]. Fifty percent of those relatives with protein C deficiency had thrombosis by the age of 50 years. This suggests that an extremely high risk of thrombosis results from a deficiency in protein C. Some years later, these families were assessed for the newly discovered factor V Leiden. The presence of factor V Leiden was found to be a common secondary defect in a high number of individuals from these families. Further investigation revealed that the risk of thrombosis was far greater for those family members carrying

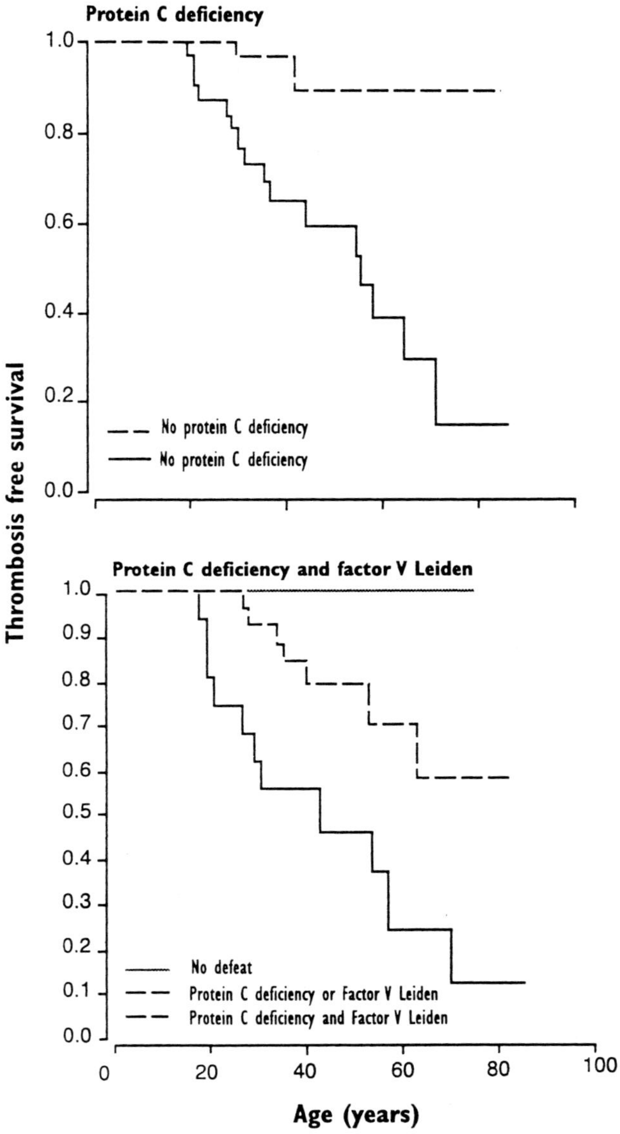

Fig. 1. Thrombosis-free survival in families with thrombophilia due to protein C deficiency (proband excluded). From [33], with permission.

both defects than for those patients carrying protein C deficiency or factor V Leiden alone [31]. From these findings it became clear that the thrombosis risk associated with protein C had been previously overestimated.

Gene–Environment Interaction

A striking example of gene–environment interaction is that relating to the use of oral contraceptives in the presence of factor V

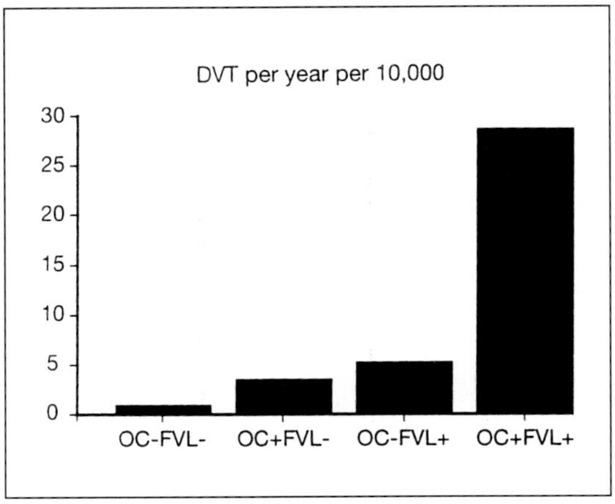

Fig. 2. Gene-environment interaction relating to the use of oral contraceptives in the presence of factor V Leiden.

Leiden, as shown in figure 2. Among unselected patients, Vandenbroucke et al. [32] revealed a synergistic effect between factor V Leiden and the use of oral contraceptives. The relative risk of thrombosis in women using oral contraceptives and carrying factor V Leiden was found to be 34.7, as compared with 6.9 for women not using oral contraceptives and carrying factor V Leiden. For women using oral contraceptives and not carrying factor V Leiden, the relative risk of thrombosis was 3.7.

Models of Thrombosis Risk

The need for a dynamic age-dependent model allowing a variety of forms of interaction of risk factors, such as additive effects or synergism, became evident when even the development of multicausal models, incorporating genetic and acquired risk factors, failed to readily explain why equal numbers of risk factors cause thrombosis in one individual and not in another, or why the same set of risk factors do not cause thrombosis in children but do so in older individuals. An example of a dynamic age-dependent model of this sort is shown in figure 3.

This model assumes that each risk factor contributes to the risk of thrombosis – this is referred to as the subject's 'thrombosis potential'. In the figure, the black lines indicate the thrombosis potential of each individual risk factor, whereas the grey lines indicate the total thrombosis potential of the individual. The figure traces the progress of a woman with factor V Leiden throughout the course of various events in her life. In the first panel, the risk factors considered are age and factor V Leiden alone. Here, the thrombosis potential, indicated by a black line, corresponds to that when no other risk factors are encountered throughout her life. The resultant overall lifetime thrombosis potential – following the insertion of an intravenous catheter while a child, the use of oral contraceptives between the age of 20 and 40, and immobilization due to a skiing accident at age 30 – follows a complicated form, and will, as a result of a combination of specific risk factors at a particular age, exceed the thrombosis threshold (shown as a broken and dotted line). As shown in the fifth panel of the figure, the thrombosis threshold is exceeded in our scenario at the age of 30 years, following immobilization, and leads to deep vein thrombosis. It is important to emphasize here that exceeding the threshold does not depend on the number of risk factors present; this same set of risk factors would not have caused thrombosis at age 20. Alternatively, if the woman had not required a plaster cast, but had continued to take oral contraceptives, thrombosis would have occurred at about the age of 50. Finally, at a greater age, the effect of age and factor V Leiden alone would have been adequate to lead to thrombosis.

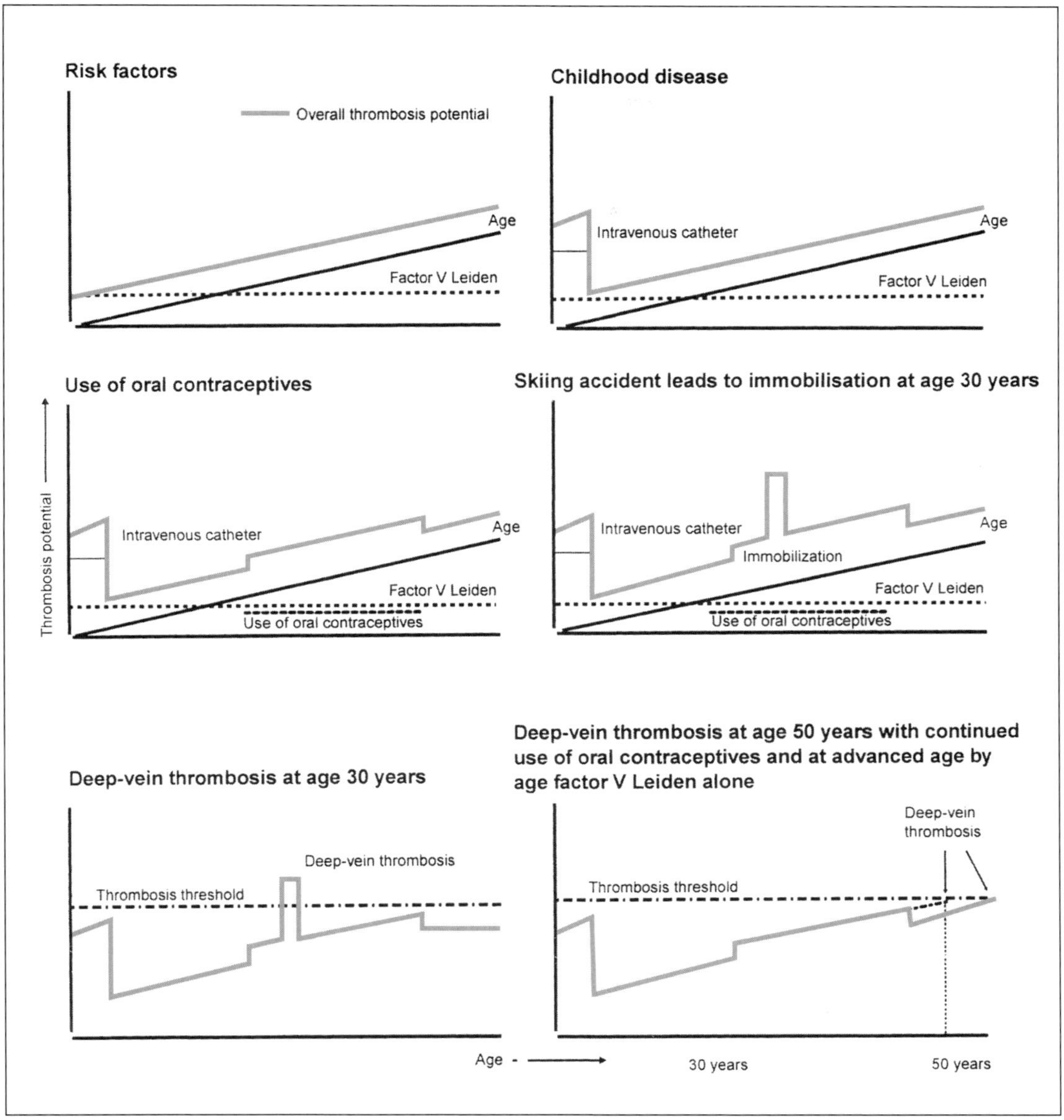

Fig. 3. Models of thrombosis risk. From Rosendaal [33].

In the model described in figure 3, it is assumed that all the risk factors considered behave in an additive fashion, i.e. without interaction. Figure 4 illustrates a refined model in which the supra-additive effects of factor V Leiden and use of oral contraceptives are taken into account. Here it can be seen that a different picture emerges regarding thrombosis potential if interactions of risk factors are taken into account in this way.

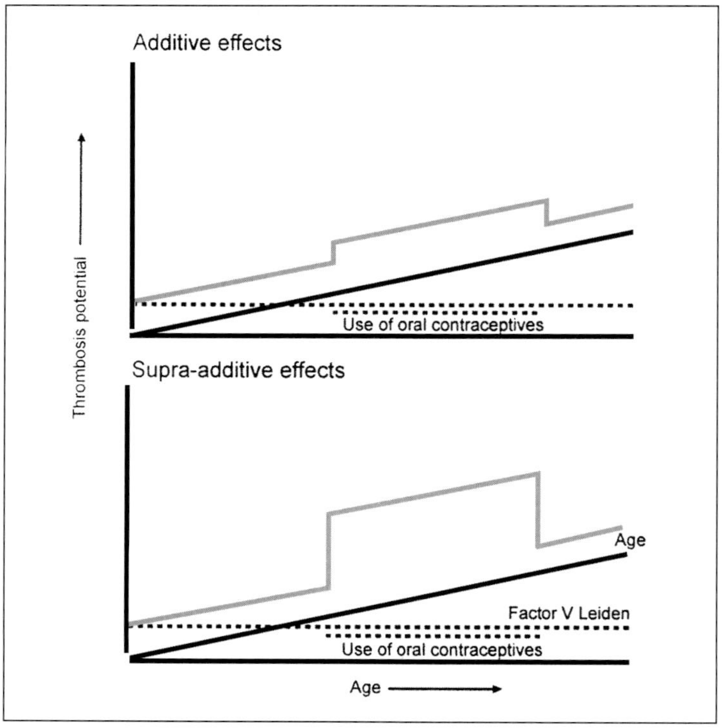

Fig. 4. Models of thrombosis risk with different interactions between factor V Leiden and use of oral contraceptives. From Rosendaal [33].

Conclusion

An important predisposing factor for venous thrombosis is age, and the disease is characterized by an interaction between genetic and acquired risk factors. Also of importance are gene–environment interactions. Individual risk can be determined by a time-dependent model in which interaction between risk factors is crucial. Such models explain why thrombosis occurs in an individual at a specific time. In the future, such models may enable the tailoring of individual risk profiles and enable guidelines to be set for prevention and prophylaxis. However, to achieve this, additional information regarding the combined effects of all possible combinations of risk factors will be required.

References

1 Egeberg O: Inherited antithrombin deficiency causing thrombophilia. Thromb Diath Haemorrh 1965;13:516–530.
2 Griffin JH, Evatt B, Zimmerman TS, Kleiss AJ, Wideman C: Deficiency of protein C in congenital thrombotic disease. J Clin Invest 1981;68:1370–1373.
3 Schwartz HP, Fischer M, Hopmeier P, Batard MA, Griffin JH: Plasma protein S deficiency in familial thrombotic disease. Blood 1984;64:1297–1300.
4 Dahlbäck B, Carlsson M, Svensson PJ: Familial thrombophilia due to a previously unrecognized mechanism characterized by poor anticoagulant response to activated protein C: Prediction of a cofactor to activated protein C. Proc Natl Acad Sci USA 1993;90:1004–1008.
5 Bertina RM, Koeleman RPC, Koster T, Rosendaal FR, Dirven RJ, de Ronde H, van der Velden PA, Reitsma PH: Mutation in blood coagulation factor V associated with resistance to activated protein C. Nature 1994;369:64–67.

6 Poort SR, Rosendaal FR, Reitsma PH, Bertina RM: A common genetic variation in the 3′-untranslated region of the prothrombin gene is associated with elevated plasma prothrombin levels and an increase in venous thrombosis. Blood 1996;88: 3698–3703.
7 Kamphuisen PW, Houwing-Duistermmaat JJ, van Houwelingen JC, Eikenboom JC, Bertina RM, Rosendaal FR: Familial clustering of factor VIII and von Willebrand factor levels. Thromb Haemost 1998;79: 323–327.
8 Koster T, Blann AD, Briët E, Vandenbroucke JP, Rosendaal FR: Role of clotting factor VIII in effect of von Willebrand factor on occurrence of deep-vein thrombosis. Lancet 1995;345:152–155.
9 Bienvenu T, Ankri A, Chadefaux B, Kamoun P: Plasma homocystein assay in the exploration of thrombosis in young subjects. Presse Méd 1991; 20:985–988.
10 Falcon CR, Cattaneo M, Panzen D, Martinelli I, Mannucci PM: High prevalence of hyperhomocyst(e)-inemia in patients with juvenile venous thrombosis. Arterioscler Thromb 1994;14:1080–1083.
11 Simioni P, Prandoni P, Burlina A, Tormene D, Sardella C, Ferrari V, Benedetti L, Girolami A: Hyperhomocysteinemia and deep-vein thrombosis: A case-control study. Thromb Haemost 1996;76:883–886.
12 Den Heijer M, Koster T, Blom HJ, Bos GM, Briet E, Reitsma PH, Vandenbroucke JP, Rosendaal FR: Hyperhomocysteinemia as a risk factor for deep-vein thrombosis. N Engl J Med 1996;334:759–762.
13 Rosendaal FR: Risk factors for venous thrombosis: Prevalence, risk and interaction. Semin Hematol 1997;34:171–187.
14 Tait RC, Walker ID, Reitsma PH, Islam SI, McCall F, Poort SR, Conkie JA, Bertina RM: Prevalence of protein C deficiency in the healthy population. Thromb Haemost 1995; 73:87–93.
15 Tait RC, Walker ID, Perry DJ, et al: Prevalence of antithrombin deficiency in the healthy population. Br J Haematol 1994;87:106–112.
16 Miletich J, Sherman L, Broze G: Absence of thrombosis in subjects with heterozygous protein C deficiency. N Engl J Med 1987;317:991–996.
17 Rosendaal FR, Koster T, Vandenbroucke JP, Reitsma PH: High risk of thrombosis in patients homozygous for factor V Leiden (activated protein C resistance). Blood 1995; 85:1504–1508.
18 Koster T, Rosendaal FR, Briët E, van der Meer FJ, Colly LP, Trienekens PH, Poort SR, Reitsma PH, Vandenbroucke JP: Protein C deficiency in a controlled series of unselected outpatients: An infrequent but clear risk factor for venous thrombosis (Leiden Thrombophilia Study). Blood 1995;85:2756–2761.
19 Rees DC, Cox M, Clegg JB: World distribution of factor V Leiden. Lancet 1995;346:1133–1134.
20 Koster T, Rosendaal FR, De Ronde H, Briët E, Vandenbroucke JP, Bertina RM: Venous thrombosis due to a poor anticoagulant response to activated protein C: Leiden Thrombophilia Study. Lancet 1993;342: 1503–1506.
21 Rosendaal FR, Doggen CJM, Zivelin A, Arruda VR, Aiach M, Siscovick DS, Hillarp A, Watzke HH, Bernardi F, Cumming AM, Preston FE, Reitsma PH: Geographic distribution of the 20210 G to A prothrombin variant. Thromb Haemost 1998;79:706–708.
22 Andrew M, Dand M, Adams M, Ali K, Anderson R, Barnard D, Bernstein M, Brisson L, Cairney B, DeSai D: Venous thromboembolic complications (VTE) in children: First analyses of the Canadian registry. Blood 1994;83:1251–1257.
23 Nuss R, Hays T, Manco-Johnson M: Childhood thrombosis. Pediatrics 1995;96:291–294.
24 Tabernero MD, Tomas JF, Alberca I, Orfao A, Lopez Borrasca A, Vicente V: Incidence and clinical characteristics of hereditary disorders associated with venous thrombosis. Am J Hematol 1991;36:249–254.
25 Griffin JH, Evatt B, Wideman C, Fernandez JA: Anticoagulant protein C pathway defective in a majority of thrombophilic patients. Blood 1993;82:1989–1993.
26 Scharrer I, Hach-Wunderle V, Heyland H, Kuhn C: Incidence of defective t-PA release in 158 unrelated young patients with venous thrombosis in comparison to PC-, PS-, AT III-, fibrinogen- and plasminogen deficiency. Thromb Haemost 1987; 58:72.
27 Ben Tal O, Zivelin A, Seligsohn U: The relative frequency of hereditary thrombotic disorders among 107 patients with thrombophilia in Israel. Thromb Haemost 1989;61:50–54.
28 Allaart CF, Poort SR, Rosendaal FR, Reitsma PH, Bertina RM, Briët E: Increased risk of venous thrombosis in carriers of protein C deficiency defect. Lancet 1993;341: 134–138.
29 Tsuda S, Reitsma P, Miletich J: Molecular defects causing heterozygous protein C deficiency in three asymptomatic kindreds. Thromb Haemost 1991;65:647.
30 Lensen RPM, Rosendaal FR, Koster T, Allart CF, de Ronde H, Vandenbroucke JP, Reitsma PH, Bertina RM: Apparent different thrombotic tendency in patients with factor V Leiden and protein C deficiency due to selection of patients. Blood 1996;88:4205–4208.
31 Koeleman BPC, Reitsma PH, Allaart CF, Bertina RM: APC-resistance as an additional risk factor for thrombosis in protein C deficient families. Blood 1994;84:1031–1035.
32 Vandenbroucke JP, Koster T, Briët E, Reitsma PH, Bertina RM, Rosendaal FR: Increased risk of venous thrombosis in oral contraceptive users who are carriers of factor V Leiden mutation. Lancet 1994;344: 1453–1457.
33 Rosendaal FR: Venous thrombosis: A multicausal disease. Lancet 1999; 353:1167–1173.

Main Paper

Hæmostasis

Haemostasis 1999;29(suppl 1):10–20

Modern Approach to Diagnosis in Patients with Suspected Deep Vein Thrombosis

Philip S. Wells[a] David R. Anderson[b]

[a]Department of Medicine and Epidemiology and Community Medicine, Ottawa Hospital and the University of Ottawa, Ottawa, Ont., and [b]Department of Medicine, Dalhousie University, Halifax, N.S., Canada

Key Words

Deep vein thrombosis · Diagnosis · Ultrasonography · D-dimer · Clinical probability · Low-molecular-weight heparin

Abstract

Deep vein thrombosis is a relatively common disease, amenable to therapy but with a potentially fatal outcome if untreated. The diagnosis can be made in most patients with the non-invasive imaging procedure ultrasonography, but limitations exist. As with all tests, there is a potential for false-positive and false-negative results. The latter are especially an issue for calf vein thrombi, and this in part has led to the concept of serial testing of the proximal venous system rather than imaging the calf. The premise of the repeat (serial) test is that only thrombi that extend to the proximal system are clinically relevant and such thrombi will be detected on the repeat test. However, despite the safety of the serial-testing concept, it is inconvenient and expensive. In the last few years, the diagnostic process has been improved by the validation of a clinical model that accurately categorizes patients as having low, moderate or high probability of deep vein thrombosis. Among the improvements this provides is the elimination of serial testing if the ultrasound is normal and the clinical probability low. The fibrin degradation product D-dimer has been demonstrated to have a high negative predictive value and has also proven

Dr. Wells and Dr. Anderson are Research Scholars of the Canadian Heart and Stroke Foundation.

KARGER

Fax + 41 61 306 12 34
E-Mail karger@karger.ch
www.karger.com

© 1999 S. Karger AG, Basel
0301–0147/99/0297–0010$17.50/0

Accessible online at:
www.karger.com/journals/hae

Dr. P. Wells
Suite 467, 737 Parkdale Avenue
Ottawa, Ont. K1Y 1J8 (Canada)

useful in diagnostic algorithms. The combination of the D-dimer with clinical model assessment will enable diagnostic-testing strategies that are more safe, effective and convenient for patients.

Copyright © 1999 S. Karger AG, Basel

Introduction

Deep vein thrombosis (DVT) affects approximately 8 in every 10,000 adults per year and ranks as the third most common cardiovascular disease, behind acute ischaemic coronary syndromes and stroke [1]. The approach to patients who present with suspected DVT is problematic for several reasons. First, if left untreated, affected patients can suffer fatal pulmonary embolism (PE). Second, attempts at using clinical diagnosis alone to predict DVT presence are not enough. Third, about 75 to 85% of patients who present with suspected DVT have non-thrombotic causes of leg pain. Finally, although anticoagulant therapy is highly effective in preventing the extension, embolization and recurrence of DVT, it is associated with an increased risk of major bleeding – over 2.4% [2] – and other potentially serious consequences such as heparin-induced thrombocytopenia. Therefore, when possible, anticoagulation should be restricted to those with confirmed DVT. For all of these reasons, it is important to diagnose DVT accurately. This will not only avoid unnecessary exposure of patients to the hazards of anticoagulant therapy, but it will also prevent many from being falsely labelled as suffering from venous thromboembolic disease.

In recent years there have been several important advances that have improved the diagnostic-testing strategies for patients with suspected DVT.

The purpose of this review is to update the reader about these recent advances and current strategies for the investigation of patients with suspected DVT.

Objective Diagnostic Testing

Before the 1970s, the diagnosis of DVT was usually made on clinical grounds. With the availability of venography, however, it became apparent that errors were made when the diagnosis of DVT was based on the clinical examination alone [3, 4]. Subsequently, the clinical diagnosis fell into such disregard that its utility was felt only to be a trigger for the consideration of the need for objective testing. Contrast venography became the reference standard diagnostic test. However, venography is expensive, uncomfortable to the patient, is technically difficult to perform, is inadequate or cannot be done in 3.6 to 10% of patients, and disagreements over the interpretation of test results occur in about 10% of cases [5, 6]. Therefore, this test is not ideal to perform routinely on all patients with suspected DVT.

In symptomatic patients, 85% of thrombi are proximal (popliteal or more proximal veins) and 15% are limited to the calf [5, 6]. This distinction is important because proximal vein thrombosis has a higher potential for causing PE and death, and also probably post-phlebitic syndrome. Pulmonary emboli are detected in approximately 50% of patients with documented proximal DVT [7], but isolated calf vein thrombosis rarely causes PE. Unfortunately, proximal extension of calf DVT occurs in 20–30% of cases [8, 9]. The above-mentioned limitations of venography and the need to detect cases of calf vein extension led to the concept of serial testing with non-invasive tests. Serial testing overcomes the lower accuracy of non-invasive tests for calf vein DVT and allows detection of clinically relevant proximal DVT. This technique was originally validated with impedance plethysmography (IPG) [10]. However, IPG is much less accurate than venous ultrasound imaging [11, 12], and therefore, in patients with suspected DVT and an initial negative study, serial testing with ultrasonography, rather than with IPG, should be undertaken.

Venous ultrasound imaging is a very accurate test for patients presenting with symptoms suspected to be caused by DVT, with lack of vein compressibility considered a positive result. A meta-analysis of studies in symptomatic patients using venography as the gold standard reported that the sensitivity of ultrasound imaging was 97% (95% CI, 96–98%) for the diagnosis of DVT involving the proximal leg veins and the specificity was 94% (95% CI, 90–98%) for all deep vein thrombi [13]. Similar accuracy rates for venous ultrasound imaging were reported in studies in which the entire proximal venous system was examined and those in which the examination was limited to the deep veins in the common femoral and the popliteal regions, extending distally to the trifurcation of the popliteal vein [13]. It should be noted that the studies to date still suggest false-positive ultrasound tests (i.e. tests interpreted as positive but found by venography to not represent acute venous thrombosis) occur in up to 6% of patients, but this fact is largely ignored [11]. Studies evaluating the accuracy of compression ultrasonography for the diagnosis of calf DVT have been relatively small and the results have been highly variable. A meta-analysis reported the sensitivity of ultrasonography for isolated calf vein thrombosis to be 73% (95% CI, 54–93%) [13]. In addition, the rates of technically inadequate analyses using ultrasonography, up to 40% in one study, were higher for calf than for proximal vein evaluation [14].

In the serial-testing strategy, patients with an initial negative study of the proximal veins have antithrombotic therapy withheld and then undergo follow-up ultrasound testing 1 week later. Patients who develop proximal extension of DVT have antithrombotic treatment initiated, whereas those with negative serial ultrasounds are presumed to not have DVT accounting for their leg symptoms. Recent large management studies by Cogo et al. [15] and Birdwell et al. [16] have shown serial ultrasound testing to be a relatively safe strategy for investigating patients with suspected DVT – those with negative serial ultrasounds had a less than 1% risk of developing symptomatic proximal DVT or PE during a 3-month follow-up period. However, serial testing has limitations.

To illustrate the main problem with serial testing, let us take a hypothetical population of 1,000 patients with suspected DVT. Assume 20% (200) will have DVT, of which 170 would be proximal and 30 calf vein. If ultrasound has a sensitivity of 97%, then 165 cases of proximal DVT will be detected, 5 cases of proximal DVT will be missed and all 30 cases of calf vein DVT will be missed with the initial test (since the calf is not imaged). If we assume nine (30%) calf clots extend and all the proximal DVT are detected 1 week later, at best 14 more cases of DVT are detected with the serial test. Note that 835 patients undergo serial testing to detect these 14 cases. Thus, serial testing is not cost-effective and is very inconvenient for most patients. Performing calf vein imaging in all patients with negative proximal examinations is likewise not desirable because it is time-consuming and the rate of inadequate scans would result in the need for additional testing in many patients. In addition, as mentioned previously, the accuracy of ultrasound is lower for calf DVT, resulting in increased false-positive and false-negative studies. Unfortunately, no prospective study has evaluated the safety of withholding anticoagulants solely on the basis of a single negative ultrasound assessment of either the proximal system alone or both the proximal and calf venous systems. Thus, it would be desirable to identify patients in whom the diagnosis of DVT could be safely excluded on the basis of a single negative ultrasonography study of the proximal venous system. Clinical assessment provides a mechanism to investigate patients according to risk.

Principle of Clinical Assessment

The concept of using pretest probability to arrive at the post-test probability of a disease with a given diagnostic test result is not unique to DVT. It is, correctly, applied to virtually all diagnoses in medicine. Although the relationship between a diagnostic test and its clinical utility is frequently described from the point of view of sensitivity and specificity reported in simple 2 × 2 tables, from a clinical point of view the primary concern is the probability of a disease in a patient with either a positive test result (positive predictive value) or a negative test result (negative predictive value). The predictive value of a test is dependent on prevalence (pretest probability). An abnormal result, using a test that has 98% sensitivity and specificity, has a positive predictive value of 99.5% when prevalence is 85%, but the predictive value is 70% when prevalence is 5%. As originally outlined by Bayes [17], the interpretation of a test result rests equally upon two factors: the initial estimate of the likelihood that a given disease is present (an estimate made in advance of the test result) and the likelihood that a given test result will occur in the patient under consideration.

Physicians experienced in the area of venous thrombosis know intuitively that if a patient has no other factors to suggest a diagnosis other than DVT, if risk factors are present, and if signs and symptoms are present, then the patient has a higher probability of having DVT. Early reports, which suggest clinical diagnosis is of no use, made the mistake of trying to predict the disease on the basis of signs and symptoms only. We incorporated signs, symptoms, risk factors and alternative diagnosis to validate a clinical scoring system that classifies patients with no previous history of DVT as having low, moderate or high probability for DVT, prior to diagnostic testing. In our original study employing clinical assessment, in which venography was used in all patients, the low, moderate and high probability groups had 5, 33 and 85%, respectively, rates of DVT [5]. Physicians also indicated their perceived pretest probability independent of the model and the prevalence was 5, 29 and 73%, but with fewer patients in the low-probability group (256 versus 301) (table 1) [18]. We simplified the model, with a regression analysis, to the following (table 1): one point is scored for the presence of paralysis, dilated superficial veins, calf swelling, entire leg swelling, cancer, immobilization, tender deep veins and pitting oedema, and minus two is scored if an alternative diagnosis that is as likely or more likely than DVT is present. These points are added together to achieve a total score. Patients with scores of 0 or less are low probability, those with scores of 1 or 2 are moderate probability, and those with scores of 3 or more are high probability.

Other investigators have studied clinical diagnosis of DVT. Landefeld and associates [19] found that five clinical findings were independently associated with the development of proximal DVT: swelling above the knee of the affected leg, swelling below the

Table 1. Clinical model for predicting pretest probability for DVT in patients with no known previous history

	Score, if present
Active cancer (treatment ongoing or within previous 6 months or palliative)	1
Paralysis, paresis or recent plaster immobilization of the lower extremities	1
Recently bedridden for > 3 days or major surgery within 4 weeks	1
Localized tenderness along the distribution of the deep venous system	1
Entire leg swollen	1
Calf swelling > 3 cm compared with asymptomatic side (measured 10 cm below tibial tuberosity)	1
Pitting oedema confined to the symptomatic leg	1
Collateral superficial veins (non-varicose)	1
Alternative diagnosis that is likely as or more likely than that of DVT	–2

Note: In patients with symptoms in both legs, the more symptomatic leg is used.

Pretest probabilities calculated as follows:

	Total points
High	≥ 3
Moderate	1 or 2
Low	≤ 0

knee, recent immobility, cancer and fever. In small numbers of patients, the prevalence of DVT was 5% if none of the findings were present, 15% if one was present and 42% if two or more were present. There are several limitations to this study, however: inpatients and outpatients were combined; the data were not collected prospectively; and 236 patients composed the derivation group and only 119 the validation set. Hence, there are wide confidence limits on the results. Nypaver et al. [20] also derived a clinical prediction score, the main limitations in this case being the small number of patients enrolled and the fact that ultrasound and clinical assessments were unblinded. If patients had no history of cancer, had less than a 3-cm difference in thigh circumference, and had had symptoms for more than 7 days, the probability of DVT was 3.3%. They were unable to derive a useful model in inpatients.

D-Dimer for the Diagnosis of Venous Thromboembolism (VTE)

Markers of thrombosis have been evaluated for their predictive value in the diagnosis of VTE. The test that has been studied most extensively and appears to be the most useful is the D-dimer [21, 22]. The D-dimer is a degradation product of a cross-linked fibrin blood clot. Levels of D-dimer are typically elevated in patients with acute VTE. Levels may also be increased in a variety of non-thrombotic disorders, including recent major surgery, haemorrhage, trauma, malignancy and sepsis. Therefore, D-dimer assays are, in general, sensitive but non-specific markers for VTE. As a result of these diagnostic characteristics, a positive D-dimer result is not useful to 'rule in' or confirm the diagnosis of VTE, rather the potential value is for a negative test result to exclude the diagnosis [21, 22]. The negative predictive value of the D-dimer increases proportionately depending upon the sensitivity of the assay and is inversely related to the prevalence of VTE in the population under study. The specificity of the particular D-dimer assay and the population under study influence the utility of the assay to exclude the diagnosis of VTE. For instance, use of a very non-specific assay or the testing of ill, hospitalized patients would be predicted to be of limited value due to the expected high false-positive rates that would be observed [21].

Several different D-dimer assays have been evaluated for the diagnosis of VTE and the accuracy of these tests varies. The most sensitive D-dimer tests are the enzyme-linked immunosorbent assays (ELISA). Bounameaux and colleagues [23] reported an ELISA D-dimer assay with a mean sensitivity of 97% and specificity of 35% for the diagnosis of DVT. Until recently, ELISA D-dimer assays were performed on microplate readers, making the assay expensive, time-consuming and not practical to be performed in most centres as an urgent diagnostic test. However, semi-quantitative and a rapid fluorescence quantitative ELISA D-dimer assays have been developed which maintain the high sensitivity of the test and have lowered the test turnaround time to less than 1 h [24, 25].

Two other D-dimer assay methods that have been evaluated as diagnostic markers for VTE are a whole-blood agglutination assay (SimpliRED) and latex agglutination plasma assays [26, 27]. These assays have the advantages that they are simple to perform, have a rapid turnaround time and are inexpensive. They are less sensitive but more specific than the ELISA assay. The sensitivity of the SimpliRED D-dimer in clinical trials has varied between 84 and 94%, whereas the latex agglutination plasma assays are less than 80% sensitive [21, 26, 27]. Prospective studies have reported that the negative predictive values of the ELISA and SimpliRED D-dimer assays exceed 95% [21, 22]. Because of its higher sensitivity, a negative ELISA D-dimer assay may be useful in itself in excluding the diagnosis of VTE. The SimpliRED, with its lower sensitivity, has been suggested as an exclusion test in patient populations identified to have a lower prevalence of VTE [28].

Diagnostic-Testing Algorithms

The simplified nine-point clinical model developed in our regression analysis has recently been employed in management studies, with a strategy as outlined in figure 1. In thrombosis referral units, we were able to demonstrate that the prevalence of DVT was 3, 17 and 75% in the groups with low, moderate and high probability, respectively. Patients at low clinical pretest probability had DVT safely excluded on the basis of a single negative ultrasound test [29]. Only 0.3% (95% CI, 0–1.7%) of patients in this subgroup developed venous thromboembolic complications in a 3-month follow-up period. About 20% of abnormal ultrasound results in this group are falsely positive and venography should be performed if the detected thrombus is small or of indeterminate age. Our study also showed that clinical diagnosis could be used to identify a subgroup of patients who were at increased risk of having a falsely negative ultrasound study. Eighteen percent of patients with a high probability of DVT and a negative ultrasound were found to have a proximal DVT by venography. However, in each case, the thrombosis involved the popliteal vein only, and arguably could have been safely detected on a serial ultrasound test a week later. This same study suggested that negative D-dimer results may be adequate to eliminate the need for diagnostic imaging of the deep veins provided the pretest probabili-

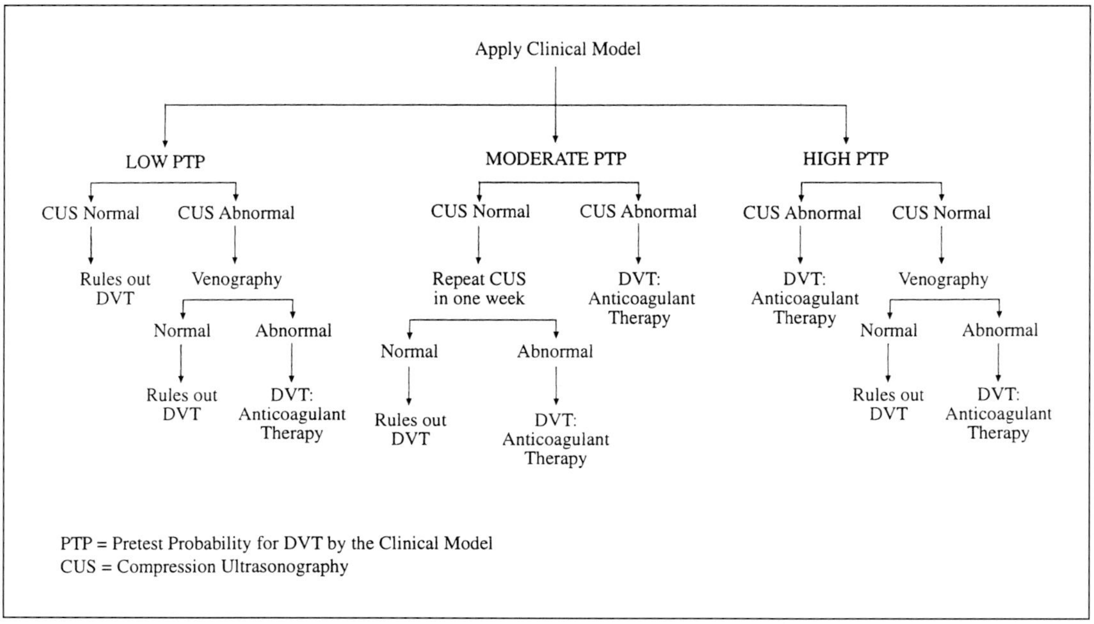

Fig. 1. Diagnostic approach in patients with suspected first episode of DVT.

ty for DVT is low [29]. We also studied the clinical model in hospitalized patients with symptoms suggestive of DVT [30]. The prevalence of DVT was 10, 21 and 76% in the groups with low, moderate and high probability, respectively. One normal ultrasound safely excluded DVT in the low-probability group, but the confidence limits on follow-up event rates extended up to 6%. More experience is required using hospitalized patients.

Clinical assessment has provided more flexibility in managing patients presenting with suspected DVT at times when radiographic imaging is not routinely available, especially in the emergency department. We have demonstrated that in patients in whom there is a moderate or high clinical suspicion of DVT, an injection of unfractionated or low-molecular-weight heparin in doses designed to treat an acute DVT is safe and can allow diagnostic imaging to be performed the following day [30–32]. Patients with low pretest probability, as assessed either by our clinical model or with the use of a sensitive D-dimer test, may have diagnostic imaging delayed for 12–24 h without the need for anticoagulant cover. Most recently, Perrier and colleagues [33] performed a management study in patients with suspected DVT in the emergency department. In patients considered to have low probability of DVT, only 2% of patients had the diagnosis made at initial testing. Perrier et al. did not use a model but used the principle of tabulating risk factors, signs, symptoms and alternative diagnosis. A potential limitation of their results is the 2.6% rate of thromboembolic events in the 3-month follow-up, as compared with 0.6% in our study employing an explicit clinical model. Furthermore, only 27% of their patients were classified as low probability, versus 55% in our series. Nonetheless, their study demon-

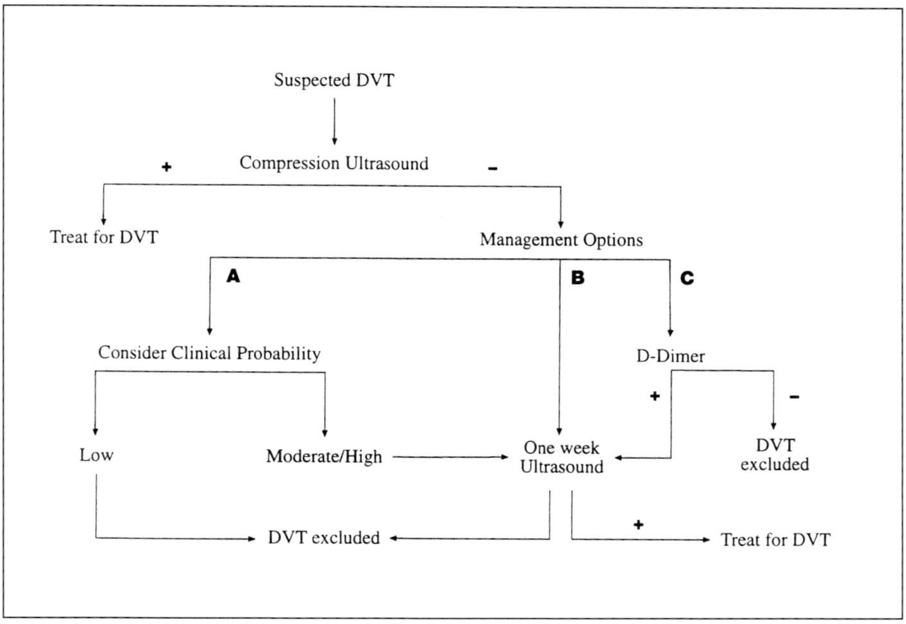

Fig. 2. Algorithm for investigation of patients with a suspected first episode of DVT.

strated that the utility of determining clinical probability can be further enhanced by also using the negative predictive value of sensitive D-dimer tests.

Ginsberg and colleagues [34] also recently evaluated the probability of DVT in patients by using D-dimer to limit the need for serial testing. They reported that among 273 patients who had a single normal result with IPG and a negative SimpliRED D-dimer result, 269 (98.5%; 95% CI, 96.3–99.6%) had no venous thromboembolic complications during the 3-month follow-up period. When this cohort was restricted to patients at low pretest probability for DVT, the negative predictive value of the D-dimer increased to 99.4%. The authors speculate that this approach would be at least as safe in patients undergoing venous ultrasound imaging, given that ultrasound is a more sensitive test than IPG for DVT.

In summary, there are at least three approaches that are reasonable to use in patients with suspected DVT. These are outlined in figure 2. It is important to emphasize, as we have described above, that a sensitive D-dimer assay must be employed, and clinical assessment should be undertaken before diagnostic testing. Venography remains an important option in selected patients, as outlined in figure 1.

Postoperative Asymptomatic Patients

The ability of physicians to determine the probability of DVT in post-operative patients without specific leg complaints is no better than by chance alone. Venous ultrasound imaging has been extensively evaluated as a screening test performed on asymptomatic patients in high-risk settings for DVT. A meta-analysis showed that the sensitivity of ultrasound imaging for proximal DVT was only 62% following total hip or knee arthroplasty and that somewhat lower sensitivity rates were observed for isolated calf vein thrombosis [35]. The sensitivity of post-operative ultrasound screening was not increased by the addition of Doppler or colour Doppler [36]. Likely explanations for the low sensitivity include small thrombus size and unpredictable thrombus location. Post-operative thrombi do not usually follow the typical anatomic distribution seen in symptomatic patients. Despite the low accuracy of ultrasonographic screening in the post-operative setting, some still advocate its use. However, a recent randomized study demonstrated that screening with venous ultrasound imaging of the proximal venous system prior to hospital discharge did not reduce the rate of subsequent symptomatic venous thromboembolic complications in patients who received warfarin prophylaxis following total hip or knee arthroplasty [37]. Based on this study, routine ultrasound screening cannot be recommended following joint arthroplasty, at least in patients receiving DVT prophylaxis. It can be concluded that symptomatic post-operative patients should undergo objective testing; whether our clinical model can select patients who require a single ultrasound test of the proximal system to rule out DVT (i.e. low-probability patients) and those in whom serial testing or venography is indicated, needs to be verified.

Summary and Conclusions

Venous ultrasound imaging, repeating the test one week later if the initial test is negative, has become the diagnostic strategy of choice in patients with suspected DVT. However, several advances in the diagnostic process have been made. First, the accuracy and the utility of the clinical diagnosis has been re-evaluated and was found to be a valuable adjunct to objective testing. Second, the fibrin degradation product the D-dimer has proven to be a sensitive and potentially useful test to exclude the diagnosis of VTE, and third, the inconvenience and cost of serial testing can be safely overcome by diagnostic-testing algorithms that incorporate the clinical assessment and/or D-dimer. Ongoing clinical trials are evaluating whether these diagnostic processes can be made even simpler and less expensive. Attempts to identify very-low-risk patients with suspected DVT, in whom imaging procedures can be avoided altogether, are already proving to be successful. Algorithms have been developed which could be useful; however, these need further validation.

References

1 Anderson FA Jr, Wheeler HB, Goldberg RJ, Hosmer DW, Patwardhan NA, Jovanovic B, Forcier A, Dalen JE: A population-based perspective of the hospital incidence and case-fatality rates of deep vein thrombosis and pulmonary embolism. The Worcester DVT Study. Arch Intern Med 1991;151:933–938.

2 Leizorovicz A, Simonneau G, Decousus H, Boissel JP: Comparison of efficacy and safety of low molecular weight heparins and unfractionated heparin in initial treatment of deep venous thrombosis: A meta-analysis. BMJ 1994;309:299–304.

3 Barnes RW, Wu KK, Hoak JC: Fallibility of the clinical diagnosis of venous thrombosis. J Am Med Assoc 1975;234:605–607.

4 Haeger K: Problems of acute venous thrombosis: The interpretation of signs and symptoms. Angiology 1969;20:219–223.

5 Wells PS, Hirsh J, Anderson DR, Lensing AWA, Foster G, Kearon C, Weitz J, D'Ovidio R, Cogo A, Prandoni P, Girolami A, Ginsberg JS: Accuracy of clinical assessment of deep-vein thrombosis. Lancet 1995; 345:1326–1330.

6 Cogo A, Lensing AWA, Prandoni P, Hirsh J: Distribution of venous thrombosis in patients with symptomatic deep vein thrombosis. Implications for simplifying the diagnostic process with compression ultrasound. Arch Intern Med 1993; 153:2777–2780.

7 Huisman MV, Buller HR, ten Cate JW, van Royen EA, Vreeken J, Kersten MJ, Bakx R: Unexpected high prevalence of silent pulmonary embolism in patients with deep vein thrombosis. Chest 1989;95:498–502.

8 Kakkar VV, Howe CT, Flanc C, Clarke MB: Natural history of postoperative deep-vein thrombosis. Lancet 1969;2:230–232.

9 Oishi CS, Grady-Benson JC, Otis SM, Colwell CW, Walker RH: The clinical course of distal deep vein thrombosis after total hip and total knee arthroplasty as determined with ultrasound. J Bone Joint Surg Am 1994;76A:1658–1663.

10 Hull RD, Hirsh J, Carter C, Jay RM, Ocketford PA, Buller HR, Turpie AG, Powers P, Kinch D, Dodd PE: Diagnostic efficiency of impedance plethysmography for clinically suspected deep vein thrombosis: A randomized trial. Ann Intern Med 1985;102:21–26.

11 Heijboer H, Buller HR, Lensing AW, Turpie AG, Colly LP, ten Cate JW: A comparison of real-time compression ultrasonography with impedance plethysmography for the diagnosis of deep-vein thrombosis in symptomatic outpatients. N Engl J Med 1993;329:1365–1369.

12 Wells PS, Hirsh J, Anderson DR, Lensing AWA, Foster G, Kearon C, Weitz J, Cogo A, Prandoni P, Minuk T, Thomson G, Benedetti L, Girolami A, Ginsberg JS: Comparison of the accuracy of impedance plethysmography and compression ultrasonography in outpatients with clinically suspected deep vein thrombosis – a two centre paired-design prospective trial. Thromb Haemost 1995;75:1423–1427.

13 Kearon C, Julian MM, Newman TE, Ginsberg JS: Noninvasive diagnosis of deep venous thrombosis. Ann Intern Med 1998;128:663–677.

14 Rose SC, Zwiebel WJ, Nelson BD, Priest DL, Knighton RA, Brown LW, Lawrence PF, Stults BM, Reading JC, Miller FJ: Symptomatic lower extremity deep venous thrombosis: Accuracy, limitations, and role of color duplex flow imaging in diagnosis. Radiology 1990;175:639–644.

15 Cogo A, Lensing AWA, Koopman MMW, Piovella F, Siragusa S, Wells PS, Villalta S, Buller H, Turpie AGG, Prandoni P: Compression ultrasonography for diagnostic management of patients with clinically suspected deep vein thrombosis: Prospective cohort study. BMJ 1998;316:17–20.

16 Birdwell BG, Raskob GE, Whitsett TL, Durica SS, Comp PC, George JN, Tytle TL, McKee PA: The clinical validity of normal compression ultrasonography in outpatients suspected of having deep venous thrombosis. Ann Intern Med 1998; 128:1–7.

17 Bayes T: An essay towards solving a problem in the doctrine of chances. Philos Trans R Soc Lond 1763;53: 370–418.

18 Wells PS, Hirsh J, Anderson DR, Lensing AWA, Foster G, Kearon C, Weitz J, D'Ovidio R, Cogo A, Prandoni P, Girolami A, Ginsberg JS: A simple clinical model for the diagnosis of deep vein thrombosis combined with impedance plethysmography: Potential for improvement in the diagnostic process. J Intern Med 1998;243:15–23.

19 Landefeld CS, McGuire E, Cohen A: Clinical findings associated with acute proximal deep vein thrombosis: A basis for quantifying clinical judgement. Am J Med 1990;88:388.

20 Nypaver TJ, Shepard AD, Kiell CS, McPharlin M, Fenn N, Ernst CB: Outpatient duplex scanning for deep vein thrombosis: Parameters predictive of a negative study result. J Vasc Surg 1993;18:821–826.

21 Lee AYY, Ginsberg JS: The role of D-dimer in the diagnosis of venous thromboembolism. Curr Opin Pulm Med 1997;3:275–279.

22 Crippa L, D'Angelo SV, Tomassini L, Rizzi B, D'Alessandro G, D'Angelo A: The utility and cost-effectiveness of D-dimer measurements in the diagnosis of deep vein thrombosis. Haematologica 1997;82:446–451.

23 Bounameaux H, de Moerloose P, Perrier A, Reber G: Plasma measurement of D-dimer as diagnostic aid in suspected venous thromboembolism: An overview. Thromb Haemost 1994;71:1–6.

24 Dale S, Gogstad GO, Brosstad F, Godal HC, Holtund J, Mark E, Brandsnes O, Borch SM: Comparison of three D-dimer assays for the diagnosis of DVT: ELISA, latex, and an immunofiltration assay (NycoCard D-dimer). Thromb Haemost 1994;71:270–274.

25 D'Angela A, D'Alessandro G, Tomassini L, Pittet JL, Dupuy G, Crippa L: Evaluation of a new rapid quantitative D-dimer assay in patients with clinically suspected deep vein thrombosis. Thomb Haemost 1996;75:412–416.

26 Elias A, Aptel I, Huc B, Chale JJ, Nguyen F, Cambus JP, Boccalon H, Boneu B: D-dimer test and diagnosis of deep vein thrombosis: A comparative study of 7 assays. Thromb Haemost 1996;76:518–522.

27 Wells PS, Brill-Edwards P, Stevens P, Panju A, Patel A, Douketis J, Ginsberg J: A novel and rapid whole-blood assay for D-dimer in patients with clinically suspected deep vein thrombosis. Circulation 1995;91:2184–2187.

28 Wells PS, Anderson DR, Bormanis J, Guy F, Mitchell M, Lewandowski B: SimpliRED D-dimer can reduce the diagnostic tests in suspected deep vein thrombosis. Lancet 1998; 351:1405–1406.

29 Wells PS, Anderson DR, Bormanis J, Guy F, Mitchell M, Gray L, Clement C, Robinson KS, Lewandowski B: Value of assessment of pretest probability of deep-vein thrombosis in clinical management. Lancet 1997;350:1795–1798.

30 Wells PS, Anderson DR, Bormanis J, Guy F, Mitchell M, Gray L, Clement C, Robinson KS, Lewandowski B: Application of a diagnostic clinical model for the management of hospitalized patients with suspected deep-vein thrombosis. Thromb Haemost 1999;81:493–497.
31 Bauld DL, Kovacs MJ: Dalteparin in emergency patients to prevent admission prior to investigation for venous thromboembolism. Am J Emerg Med 1999;17:11–15.
32 Anderson DR, Wells PS, Stiell I, MacLeod B, Simms M, Gray L, Robinson S, Bormanis J, Mitchell M, Lewandowski B, Flowerdew G: Thrombosis in the emergency department: Use of a clinical diagnosis model to safely avoid the need for urgent radiological investigation. Arch Intern Med 1999;159:477–482.
33 Perrier A, Desmarais S, Miron MJ, de Moerloose P, Lepage R, Slosman D, Didier D, Unger PF, Patenaude JV, Bounameaux H: Non-invasive diagnosis of venous thromboembolism in outpatients. Lancet 1999; 353:190–195.
34 Ginsberg JS, Kearon C, Douketis J, Turpie AG, Brill-Edwards P, Stevens P, Panju A, Crowther M, Andrew M, Massicotte P, Hirsh J, Weitz J: The use of D-dimer testing and impedance plethysmographic examination in patients with clinical indications of deep vein thrombosis. Arch Intern Med 1997;157: 1077–1081.
35 Wells PS, Lensing AW, Davidson BL, Prins MH, Hirsh J: Accuracy of ultrasound for the diagnosis of deep venous thrombosis in asymptomatic patients after orthopedic surgery. A meta-analysis. Ann Intern Med 1995;122:47–53.
36 Lensing AW, Doris CI, McGrath FP, Cogo A, Sabine MJ, Ginsberg J, Prandoni P, Turpie AG, Hirsh J: A comparison of compression ultrasound with color Doppler ultrasound for the diagnosis of symptomless postoperative deep vein thrombosis. Arch Intern Med 1997;157: 765–768.
37 Robinson KS, Anderson DR, Gross M, Petrie D, Leighton R, Stanish W, Alexander D, Mitchell M, Flemming B, Gent M: Ultrasonographic screening before hospital discharge for deep venous thrombosis after arthroplasty: The post-arthroplasty screening study. Ann Intern Med 1997;127:439–445.

Main Paper

Hæmostasis

Haemostasis 1999;29(suppl 1):21–22

Modern Strategy for Diagnosis and Treatment of Pulmonary Embolism

J.P. Laaban

Department of Pneumology and Intensive Care, Hôtel-Dieu Hospital, Paris, France

Key Words

Pulmonary embolism · Venous thromboembolism · Heparin · Thrombolytic · Thoracic computed tomodensitometry · Lung scintigraphy

Abstract

Various techniques are available for the diagnosis of pulmonary embolism (PE), including pulmonary angiography, perfusion-ventilation lung scanning, D-dimer measurement, venous ultrasonography and, most recently, helical computerized tomography of the chest. The advantages and disadvantages of these techniques, used alone or in combination, are briefly discussed. Studies have indicated that treatment with low-molecular-weight heparin (LMWH), as well as being more convenient to administer, is as safe and effective as standard heparin therapy in acute PE. However, the efficacy and safety of LMWH in patients with acute PE and haemodynamic instability requires verification. Finally, the indications of inferior vena caval filters and thrombolytic therapy are outlined.

Copyright © 1999 S. Karger AG, Basel

Pulmonary angiography is the gold standard for the diagnosis of pulmonary embolism (PE), but has the drawback of being invasive. Perfusion-ventilation lung scan is inconclusive in 70% of patients with suspicion of PE and should be associated with other non-invasive tests. The measurement of plasma D-dimers using a rapid enzyme-linked immunosorbent assay (Vidas test) could be very useful because this test has a very high sensitivity (98%) for the diagnosis of acute venous thromboembolism and it is automated and quick to perform (35 min). In patients with inconclusive lung scans, the detection of deep vein thrombosis using venous ultrasonography or impedance plethysmography is sufficient to start anticoagulant therapy, but a negative leg study does not rule out PE. Non-invasive strategies combining lung scan, D-dimer measurement, venous ultrasonography and clinical probability have been validated [1], but these strategies are not suitable for patients with suspicion of massive PE.

Helical computerized tomography (CT) of the chest is a new imaging technique that can be very useful for the diagnosis of PE [2]. Studies comparing helical CT scan with pulmonary angiography have shown that CT

KARGER

Fax + 41 61 306 12 34
E-Mail karger@karger.ch
www.karger.com

© 1999 S. Karger AG, Basel
0301–0147/99/0297–0021$17.50/0

Accessible online at:
www.karger.com/journals/hae

Prof. J.P. Laaban
Department of Pneumology and Intensive Care
Hôtel-Dieu Hospital, 1, Place du Parvis, Notre-Dame
F–75181 Paris Cedex 04 (France)

scan has very high sensitivity and specificity for the diagnosis of proximal PE. Furthermore, it is widely available and minimally invasive, with very few contraindications, a low rate of technical failure and a very good inter-observer agreement. The main drawback of the technique is its very low sensitivity for the diagnosis of subsegmental PE, so that a normal CT scan cannot rule out PE. However, isolated subsegmental pulmonary emboli are very rare and their clinical importance is controversial. Preliminary data from a prospective study performed in our department suggest that a non-invasive strategy using helical CT scan is accurate to diagnose and rule out massive PE without the need for pulmonary angiography.

In acute PE, the THESEE (Tinzaparine ou Heparine Standard: Evaluations dans l'Embolie Pulmonaire) study [3] showed that the rates of death, recurrent venous thromboembolism and major bleeding did not significantly differ between the patients receiving low-molecular-weight heparin (LMWH; tinzaparin given subcutaneously once-daily in a fixed dose) and those receiving unfractionated heparin (UFH; given intravenously in an adjusted dose). Comparable results have been reported by the Columbus Investigators with reviparin [4]. It appears that LMWH is as effective and safe as UFH in acute PE, while being more convenient (one or two injections daily instead of continuous intravenous infusion, with no need for laboratory monitoring). However, no data are available on the efficacy and safety of LMWH in patients suffering from acute PE with haemodynamic instability.

The indications of inferior vena caval filters [5] should be limited. They include: contraindication of anticoagulation, complication (major bleeding) of anticoagulation, recurrent PE despite adequate anticoagulation, surgical pulmonary embolectomy, and chronic pulmonary hypertension related to recurrent PE.

The indications of thrombolytic therapy are massive PE with shock or echocardiographic evidence of right ventricular dysfunction. Urokinase, streptokinase or tissue plasminogen activator (t-PA) can be used, but a more rapid haemodynamic improvement has been reported with t-PA (100 mg infusion over 2 h). However, the beneficial effects of thrombolytic therapy on short-term mortality or on subsequent pulmonary hypertension have not yet been demonstrated.

References

1 Perrier A, Bounameaux H, Morabia A , de Moerloose PH, Slosman D, Didier D, Unger PF, Junod A: Diagnosis of pulmonary embolism by a decision analysis-based strategy including clinical probability, D-dimer levels, and ultrasonography: A management study. Arch Intern Med 1996;156:531–536.

2 Rémy-Jardin M, Rémy J, Wattine L, Giraud F: Central pulmonary thromboembolism: Diagnosis with spiral volumetric CT with the single-breath-hold technique. Comparison with pulmonary angiography. Radiology 1992;185:381–387.

3 Simonneau G, Sors H, Charbonnier B, Page Y, Laaban JP, Azarian R, Laurent M, Hirsch JL, Ferrari E, Bosson JL, Mottier D, Beau B for the THESEE Study group: A comparison of low-molecular-weight heparin with unfractionated heparin for acute pulmonary embolism. N Engl J Med 1997;337:663–669.

4 The Columbus Investigators: Low-molecular-weight heparin in the treatment of patients with venous thromboembolism. N Engl J Med 1998;338:409–415.

5 Decousus H, Leizorovicz A, Parent F, Page Y, Tardy B, Girard PH, Laporte S, Faivre R, Charbonnier B, Barral FG, Huet Y, Simonneau G for the Prévention du Risque d'Embolie Pulmonaire par Interruption Cave Study Group: A clinical trial of vena caval filters in the prevention of pulmonary embolism in patients with proximal deep-vein thrombosis. Prévention du Risque d'Embolie Pulmonaire par Interruption Cave Study Group. N Engl J Med 1998; 338:409–415.

Main Paper

Hæmostasis

Haemostasis 1999;29(suppl 1):23–31

Extended Prophylaxis against Venous Thromboembolism following Total Hip and Knee Replacement

Russell D. Hull Graham F. Pineo

Thrombosis Research Unit, University of Calgary, Calgary, Alta., Canada

Key Words

Venous thromboembolism · Low-molecular-weight heparin · Thromboprophylaxis · Orthopaedic

Abstract

The recently reported reductions in the incidence of post-operative venous thromboembolism (VTE) are related to the widespread use of prophylactic anticoagulants. Many uncertainties remain with regard to the most effective ways to use thromboprophylaxis, however. The trend towards shorter hospital stays means that patients may receive less than the recommended 7–10 days of prophylaxis. Prolonged periods of thromboprophylaxis may be beneficial for patients at high risk of post-operative VTE, such as those undergoing major orthopaedic surgery. The relative rarity of symptomatic deep vein thrombosis and pulmonary embolism means that very large patient populations are required for studies that rely on clinical endpoints, but studies using venographic endpoints have shown 28–35 days of prophylaxis with low-molecular-weight heparin to be more effective than 10–14 days. Other factors that may influence the efficacy of thromboprophylaxis include the timing of the first injection and the choice of agent.

Copyright © 1999 S. Karger AG, Basel

Introduction

Patients undergoing major orthopaedic surgery have a relatively high risk of post-operative venous thromboembolism (VTE) [1, 2]. Thromboprophylaxis has traditionally ended when the patient leaves hospital, but there is evidence that the risk of VTE extends well beyond the immediate post-operative period [3]. In addition, the current trend to-

KARGER

Fax + 41 61 306 12 34
E-Mail karger@karger.ch
www.karger.com

© 1999 S. Karger AG, Basel
0301–0147/99/0297–0023$17.50/0

Accessible online at:
www.karger.com/journals/hae

Dr. R. Hull
Thrombosis Research Unit, University of Calgary
601 South Tower-Foothills Hospital
1403–29 Street NW
Calgary, Alta. T2N 2T9 (Canada)

Table 1. Levels of evidence used in previous antithrombotic consensus conference report

Level of evidence	Grade of recommendation
Level I	*Grade A*
Level I	Results come from a single RCT in which the lower limit of the CI for the treatment effect exceeds the minimal clinically important benefit
Level I +	Results come from a meta-analysis of RCTs in which the treatment effects from individual studies are consistent, and the lower limit of the CI for the treatment effect exceeds the minimal clinically important benefit
Level I –	Results come from a meta-analysis of RCTs in which the treatment effects from individual studies are widely disparate, but the lower limit of the CI for the treatment effect still exceeds the minimal clinically important benefit
Level II	*Grade B*
Level II	Results come from a single RCT in which the CI for the treatment effect overlaps the minimal clinically important benefit
Level II +	Results come from a meta-analysis of RCTs in which the treatment effects from individual studies are consistent, and the CI for the treatment effect overlaps the minimal clinically important benefit
Level II –	Results come from a meta-analysis of RCTs in which the treatment effects from individual studies are widely disparate, and the CI for the treatment effect overlaps the minimal clinically important benefit
Level III	*Grade C* Results come from non-randomized concurrent cohort studies
Level IV	*Grade C* Results come from non-randomized historic cohort studies
Level V	*Grade C* Results come from case series

Reprinted with permission from Clagget et al. Chest 1998;114:531S–560S.

wards shorter hospital admissions reduces the duration of thromboprophylaxis and further increases the likelihood of VTE following discharge. The introduction of low-molecular-weight heparins (LMWHs), which can be self-administered by patients, means that a practical alternative to oral anticoagulants is now available for outpatient use.

This article considers the evidence that longer periods of thromboprophylaxis are of benefit to patients. It is based on data that meet the criteria of level-1 evidence, i.e. randomized trials in which the lower limit of the confidence interval for the treatment effect exceeds the minimal clinically important benefit (table 1). This approach was used by the American College of Chest Physicians (ACCP) in drawing up their 1998 Consensus Report [4]. Meta-analyses have been shown to have limitations [5] and are consequently not included in this article.

Relevance of Trial Design

Key issues in thromboprophylaxis concern trial design and the choice of endpoints. Studies based on clinical event rates have obvious clinical relevance, and if a significant benefit can be shown for a therapy or procedure, then the results are incontrovertible. However, the accuracy of clinical diagnosis of VTE is poor [6], and since routine thromboprophylaxis has become widespread following total hip-joint replacement, fatal PE is, fortunately, an uncommon event [7, 8]. Mortality rates in patients receiving thromboprophylaxis in clinical trials who have undergone total hip or knee replacement are currently in the region of 0.7%. Limited data from autopsy studies in medical and surgical patients [9] or following total hip replacement [10] indicate that fatal PE remains a significant clinical problem.

Data from studies which rely on clinical endpoints have been used in North America to support the claim that current thromboprophylactic regimens have reduced patient mortality from PE to very low rates (see below) and that there is therefore no need to provide extended prophylaxis [11–14]. However, this argument fails to recognize that the small sample size of the studies makes it difficult to detect statistically significant differences in the incidence of fatal PE.

It is now ethically unacceptable to perform placebo-controlled trials of thromboprophylaxis in major orthopaedic surgery. Trials using an active comparator require very large patient populations, in the region of 40,000, to detect a difference in the incidence of fatal PE. Studies of this size have not yet been performed, and because of the cost implications, the implementation of such studies would be very difficult.

An alternative approach is for all patients taking part in clinical trials to undergo screening venography. Studies using routine venography to detect proximal and calf DVT have consistently found a much higher incidence of VTE than studies relying on clinical diagnosis [2, 15, 16]. The majority of asymptomatic isolated calf DVTs resolve spontaneously but a proportion will propagate proximally. Fatal PE may typically follow an asymptomatic proximal DVT. Clinical trials that include venography as a screening procedure allow identification of all DVTs and offer the great advantage that smaller patient populations can be used to make meaningful comparisons of different agents and treatment regimens. Table 2 categorizes the studies according to the level of evidence identified. The studies using clinical endpoints and those using venographic endpoints are described in the following sections (tables 3–7).

Table 2. Summary of trial classification according to level of evidence identified

Author	Level classification
Mohr et al., 1993 [11]	III
Robinson et al., 1997 [12]	III
Lieberman et al., 1997 [13]	III
Leclerc et al., 1988 [14]	III
Colwell et al., 1999 [15]	III
Lassen et al., 1991 [16]	I
Hull et al., 1990 [17]	I
Bergqvist et al., 1996 [18]	I
Planes et al., 1996 [19]	I
Dahl et al., 1997 [20]	I
Lassen et al., 1998 [21]	I

Clinical Endpoints or Non-Invasive Screening

Studies in orthopaedic patients using symptomatic VTE as an endpoint have generally concluded that when some form of thromboprophylaxis is used, the incidence is very low (table 3). Mohr et al. [11] found that there was little difference between the incidence of VTE with regimens including LMWH, adjusted-dose heparin and adjusted-dose warfarin. Robinson and colleagues [12] performed

Table 3. Prevalence of symptomatic DVT and PE at 84–90 days among cohort studies of all in-hospital prophylaxis, after total hip replacement (THR) or total knee replacement (TKR) surgery

Author	Operation	No.	Prophylaxis type, in hospital	Duration of prophylaxis, days	Symptomatic DVT or PE, n (%)	Fatal PE, n (%)
Mohr et al. [11]	THR	638	Warfarin	10–14	6 (0.9)	0
Robinson et al. [12]	THR	249	Warfarin	9.8	3 (1.2)	0
	TKR	257	Warfarin	9.8	2 (0.8)	0
Lieberman et al. [13]	THR	1,099	Warfarin	15	17 (1.2)	1 (0.1)
Leclerc et al. [14]	THR	1,142	LMWH	9	49 (4.3)	0
	TKR	842	LMWH	9	33 (3.9)	3 (0.4)
Colwell et al. [15]	THR	1,516	LMWH	7.3	3.7	2 (0.001)*
	THR	1,495	Warfarin	7.3	4.5	2 (0.001)**

* One autopsy-proven, one probable PE; ** two probable PE.
Modified with permission from Colwell et al. [15].

a randomized prospective trial to find the incidence of VTE after hip and knee replacement surgery. Patients received thromboprophylaxis with warfarin for a mean period of 9.8 days before hospital discharge. The study included 249 patients undergoing hip replacement and 257 undergoing knee replacement. During the 3-month follow-up period, the incidence of symptomatic DVT or PE was 1.2% among hip-replacement patients and 0.8% among knee-replacement patients. There were no fatal PEs in either group. The incidence of VTE in patients who underwent routine ultrasound screening before hospital discharge was 1.2% after hip replacement and 0.4% after knee replacement. The authors therefore concluded that ultrasound screening was not a worthwhile procedure. On the basis of this trial, it would be reasonable to conclude that the incidence of late VTE was low and that extended prophylaxis was of no clinical value.

Lieberman et al. [13] examined 1,099 patients undergoing total hip replacement, all of whom received a mean of 15 days of warfarin prophylaxis. Follow-up, as in the other studies, was for 3 months. Symptomatic VTE occurred in 17 patients (1.2%) and there was one fatal PE. In another specifically designed study, Leclerc et al. [14] enrolled 1,984 patients undergoing hip or knee replacement. Patients received thromboprophylaxis with the LMWH enoxaparin (30 mg twice daily) for up to 14 days (mean 9 days), starting 6–24 h after surgery. The incidence of clinically suspected VTE, confirmed by objective testing, was 4.1% at 12 weeks (4.3% after hip replacement and 3.9% after knee replacement). Events were equally divided into those occurring during and after the period of prophylaxis (2.1 and 2.0%, respectively). There were three fatal PEs during hospitalization, all of which occurred in patients who had undergone knee replacement (0.4%).

In the most recent study by Colwell et al. [15] in 3,011 patients undergoing total hip replacement, 1,516 patients received LMWH

Table 4. Effect of extended thromboprophylaxis on the incidence of venographic DVT and PE after total hip replacement [18]

	Prophylaxis (in hospital/out of hospital)		p value
	enoxaparin/ enoxaparin	enoxaparin/ placebo	
Patients	117	116	
Duration of prophylaxis, days (in hospital/out of hospital)	11/19	10/18	
Proximal DVT	8 (6.8%)	28 (24.1%)	<0.001
Distal DVT	13 (11.1%)	15 (12.9%)	NS
Total DVT	21 (17.9%)	43 (37.0%)	<0.001
Non-fatal PE	0	2 (1.7%)	
Fatal PE	0	0	

(enoxaparin) 30 mg twice daily and 1,495 patients received warfarin started the night before or the night of surgery for a mean of 7.3 days. The cumulative incidence of DVT and PE at 90 days was 3.7 and 4.5 for the enoxaparin and warfarin groups, respectively. During the out-of-hospital phase, four patients died of suspected or proven PE: two in the enoxaparin group (one autopsy-proven) and two in the warfarin group. The results of the five studies using clinical endpoints or non-invasive screening are summarized in table 3.

Venographically Controlled Trials

Bergqvist et al. [18] examined the effects of thromboprophylaxis with enoxaparin for a total period of 30 days in patients undergoing total hip replacement. The control group received enoxaparin during hospital admission (10–11 days), followed by placebo to day 30. All patients underwent routine venography 19–23 days after hospital discharge.

Adequate venographic data were available from 233 patients. The total incidence of VTE was 37% among patients receiving in-hospital enoxaparin only, compared with 18% among patients receiving extended prophylaxis ($p < 0.001$) (table 4). The incidence of proximal DVT was also significantly lower in patients receiving extended thromboprophylaxis. There were no PEs among patients receiving extended thromboprophylaxis, although PE was diagnosed in two patients in the placebo group. Patients receiving prolonged enoxaparin had a higher incidence of injection-site haematoma, but there were no major haemorrhages. Thus, this study indicates that longer periods of thromboprophylaxis offer patients additional protection from VTE.

Similar findings have been reported by others. In the study by Planes et al. [19], a population of elective-hip-replacement patients, who had all received prophylactic enoxaparin (40 mg/day) for 14 days, underwent bilateral venography at the time of hospital discharge. Patients with no evidence of DVT were then randomized to receive continued enoxaparin (40 mg/day) or placebo, for a further 21 days. Venography was repeated at the end of the study or earlier if clinically indicated. Adequate data were obtained from 173 patients. The total incidence of

Table 5. Effect of extended prophylaxis in patients with no venographic evidence of DVT at hospital discharge after total hip replacement [19]. All patients had previously received 14 days of inpatient thromboprophylaxis with enoxaparin, 40 mg daily

	Enoxaparin 40 mg/day	Placebo	p value
Patients	85	88	
Duration of outpatient prophylaxis (days)	21	21	
Proximal DVT	5 (5.9%)	7 (8.0%)	NS
Distal DVT	1 (1.2%)	10 (11.4%)	0.006
Total DVT	6 (7.1%)	17 (19.3%)	0.018
PE	0	0	

Table 6. Effect of extended prophylaxis (35 days in total) in patients with no venographic evidence of proximal DVT at hospital discharge (7 days post-operatively) after total hip replacement [20]

	Out of hospital	
	dalteparin	placebo
Patients	93	89
Duration of treatment out of hospital (days)	28	28
Venographic DVT (Day 7–35)		
Proximal	4 (4.3%)	9 (10.1%)
Distal	7 (7.5%)	14 (15.7%)
Total	11 (11.8%)	23 (25.8%) p = 0.017
Clinical PE		
Total	0	3 (2.9%)
Fatal	0	1 (1.0%)

VTE was 7.1% among patients who had received prolonged enoxaparin, compared with 19.3% among the placebo group (p = 0.018; table 5). No cases of PE were reported. This study thus supports the findings of Bergqvist et al. [18].

Dahl et al. [20] have examined prolonged thromboprophylaxis with dalteparin, dextran and elastic stockings. At day 7, all patients underwent bilateral venography, perfusion-ventilation lung scanning and chest X-ray. Only those with no evidence of proximal DVT entered the next phase of the study. Eligible patients were randomized into two groups: one group continued dalteparin, 5,000 IU daily, for 28 days, and the second group received placebo treatment. Screening tests for VTE were then repeated. During the period to day 35, the incidence of DVT was 31.7% in the placebo-treated group compared with 19.3% in the dalteparin-treated group (p = 0.034; table 6). Three patients (2.9%) treated with placebo suffered PE, one of which was fatal. There were no cases of PE in the dalteparin group.

In a study by Lassen et al. [21], lower rates of DVT were reported, but the trend was similar. After 7 days of standard thromboprophylaxis with dalteparin, patients were randomized: they either continued dalteparin, 5,000 IU

Table 7. Effect of extended prophylaxis on the incidence of DVT and PE at 35 days in patients undergoing total hip replacement [21]

	Prophylaxis (in hospital/out of hospital)	
	dalteparin/ dalteparin	dalteparin/ placebo
Patients	113	102
Duration of prophylaxis, days (in hospital/out of hospital)	7/28	7/28
Venographic DVT		
Proximal	1 (0.9%)	5 (5.0%), p = 0.076
Distal	4 (3.5%)	7 (6.8%)
Total	5 (4.4%)	12 (11.8%), p = 0.039
PE	0	2

Table 8. Effect of timing of first dose of prophylactic LMWH (enoxaparin) on venographic DVT incidence at 3 months in patients undergoing total hip replacement [22]

	Preoperative	Post-operative	p value
Patients	329	658	
Proximal DVT	22 (6.7%)	34 (5.2%)	NS
Distal DVT	11 (3.3%)	67 (10.2%)	<0.001
Total DVT	33 (10.0%)	101 (15.3%)	0.023

daily, for a further 28 days, or received placebo. All patients underwent bilateral venography at the end of the study. The total DVT rate in the placebo group was 11.8%, compared with 4.4% in the patients receiving prolonged dalteparin (p = 0.039) (table 7). Five patients (5.0%) receiving placebo developed proximal DVT, compared with only one patient (0.9%) receiving prolonged dalteparin (p = 0.076). There were two non-fatal cases of PE, both in patients receiving placebo.

Timing of Thromboprophylaxis

Concerns about the risk of perioperative bleeding, particularly in association with spinal anaesthesia, have meant that the usual practice in North America is to start thromboprophylaxis up to 24 h post-operatively. By contrast, in Europe it is usual to start thromboprophylaxis 12 h preoperatively. These different regimens have made it difficult to compare the results of trials from North America and Europe, and no direct comparisons of the two approaches have yet been undertaken. A recently published meta-analysis reviewed the inpatient phase of thromboprophylactic studies using enoxaparin [22]. Comparisons were made across trials, and may thus have been influenced by factors other than timing, but the results indicate that preoperative thromboprophylaxis may offer a significant advantage over a post-operative start (see table 8). The frequency of major bleeding was less for the group receiving pre-operatively initiated LMWH than for the group receiving post-operatively initiated LMWH (0.9 vs. 3.5%, p = 0.01). Adequate data across the trials were reported for age, sex, duration of prophylaxis, and the interval between the operation and venography. The outcomes observed cannot be attributed to differences in the reported values in the key variables. Comorbid factors were not consistently reported, and, thus, differences in comorbidity may have influenced the observed outcomes. Variations in the centres in which the trials were conducted and differences in clinical practice also may have contributed to the observed outcomes. Although findings from a meta-analysis cannot be regarded as conclusive, these data fit with our knowledge of the pathogenesis of VTE and provide a hypothesis for further testing in future trials.

In the North American Fragmin Trial (NAFT), patients were randomized to the LMWH dalteparin, started within 2 h preoperatively or 6 h post-operatively, and continued for 35 days [23, 24]. The initial dose of 2,500 IU was followed by 5,000 IU daily. Bilateral venograms were performed at 6 ± 2 days and 35 ± 3 days; only those with negative venograms at 6 ± 2 days continued into the extended prophylaxis study. This study compared the efficacy of LMWH started preoperatively or post-operatively with warfarin and assessed the need for extended prophylaxis. The results of this study will be reported later this year.

Discussion

Despite wide variations in event rates, the results from level-1 trials using venographic endpoints consistently show a lower incidence of VTE with prolonged thromboprophylaxis. Centre-to-centre variability is high in clinical trials of thromboprophylaxis following total hip replacement. Trends towards a lower rate with prolonged thromboprophylaxis are therefore more relevant than the absolute event rates reported in each trial.

The size of the study population appears to be critical in these studies, and it is likely that much larger trials would produce more conclusive results. The choice of thromboprophylactic agent and the timing of the initiation of prophylaxis may also be critical.

Most trials of thromboprophylaxis have been based on a treatment period of 9–10 days, and the current ACCP recommendations are for 7–10 days of treatment [25]. However, hospital stays are usually shorter than this: 4–5 days after hip replacement is now commonplace in the United States. These data suggest that, at the very least, we should be offering out-of-hospital prophylaxis for a short period in order to ensure that adequate primary thromboprophylaxis has been achieved.

For high-risk patients, it appears that the period of thromboprophylaxis should be extended to 1 month. The ACCP recommended that a total of 29–35 days of thromboprophylaxis with LMWH may offer additional protection [25]. Relatively few data on prolonged thromboprophylaxis are currently available, and, in recognition of the slight uncertainty that still surrounds this area with respect to the risk-benefit ratio and cost implication, the ACCP have made this a level-A2 recommendation. However, with the results emerging from clinical trials that meet the criteria for level-1 data, we may see the status of this recommendation upgraded.

References

1 Kakkar VV, Howe CT, Flank C, Clarke MB: Natural history of postoperative deep-vein thrombosis. Lancet 1969;ii:230–232.
2 Turpie AGG, Levine M, Hirsh J, Carter CJ, Jay RM, Powers PJ, Andrew M, Hull RD, Gent M: A randomized controlled trial of a low-molecular-weight heparin (enoxaparin) to prevent deep-vein thrombosis in patients undergoing elective hip surgery. N Engl J Med 1986;315: 925–929.
3 Scurr JH: How long after surgery does the risk of thromboembolism persist? Acta Chir Scand Suppl 1990;556:22–24.
4 Guyatt GH, Cook DJ, Sacket DL, Eckman M, Pauker S: Grades of recommendation for antithrombotic agents. Chest 1998;114:441S–444S.
5 LeLorier J, Gregoire G, Benhaddad A, Lapierre J, Derderian F: Discrepancies between meta-analyses and subsequent large randomized, controlled trials. N Engl J Med 1997; 337:536–542.
6 Hull RD, Pineo GF: Clinical features of deep venous thrombosis; in Hull RD, Raskob GE, Pineo GF (eds): Venous Thromboembolism: An Evidence Based Atlas. Amonk, Futura Publishing, 1996, pp 87–91.
7 Seagroatt V, Tan HS, Goldacre M, Bulstrode C, Nugent I, Gill L: Elective total hip replacement: Incidence emergency readmission rate, and post-operative mortality. BMJ 1991;303:1431–1435.
8 Warwick D, Williams MH, Bannister GC: Death and thromboembolic disease after total hip replacement. J Bone Joint Surg Br 1995;77:6–10.
9 Linbald B, Eriksson BT, Bergqvist D: Autopsy-verified pulmonary embolism in a surgical department: Analysis of the period from 1951 to 1988. Br J Surg 1991;78:849–852.
10 Campling EA, Devlin HB, Hoile RW, Lunn JN: The report of the National Confidential Enquiry into Perioperative Deaths 1991/1992. London, The National Confidential Enquiry into Perioperative Deaths, 1993.
11 Mohr DN, Silverstein MD, Murtaugh PA, Harrison JM: Prophylactic agents for venous thrombosis in elective hip surgery. Arch Intern Med 1993;153:2221–2228.
12 Robinson KS, Anderson D, Gross M, Petrie D, Leighton R, Stanish W, Alexander D, Mitchell M, Flemming B, Gent M: Ultrasonographic screening before hospital discharge for deep venous thrombosis after arthroplasty: The Post-Arthroplasty Screening Study. Ann Intern Med 1997;127:439–445.
13 Lieberman JR, Wollaeger J, Dorey F, Thomas BJ, Kilgus DJ, Grecula MJ, Finerman GA, Amstutz HC: The efficacy of prophylaxis with low-dose warfarin for prevention of pulmonary embolism following total hip arthroplasty. J Bone Joint Surg Am 1997;79:319–325.
14 Leclerc J, Gent M, Hirsh J, Geerts WH, Ginsberg JS: The incidence of symptomatic venous thromboembolism during and after prophylaxis with enoxaparin. A multi-institutional cohort study of patients who underwent hip or knee arthroplasty. Arch Intern Med 1988;158:873–878.
15 Colwell CW Jr, Collis DK, Paulson R, McCutchen JW, Bigler GT, Lutz S, Hardwick ME: Comparison of enoxaparin and warfarin for the prevention of venous thromboembolic disease after total hip arthroplasty. Evaluation during hospitalization and three months after discharge. J Bone Joint Surg Am 1999;81:932–940.
16 Lassen M, Borris LC, Christiansen HM, Boll KL, Eiskjaer SP, Nielsen BW, Schott P, Olsen AD, Rodenberg JC, Lucht U: Prevention of thromboembolism in 190 hip arthroplasties: comparison of LMW heparin and placebo. Acta Orthop Scand 1991;62:33–38.
17 Hull RD, Raskob GE, Gent M, McLoughlin D, Julian D, Smith FCM, Dale NI, Reed-Davis R, Lofthouse RN, Anderson C: Effectiveness of intermittent pneumatic leg compression for preventing DVT after total hip replacement. J Am Med Assoc 1990;263:2313–2317.
18 Bergqvist D, Benoni G, Bjorgell O, Fredin H, Hedlundh U, Nicolas S, Nillson P, Nylander G: Low-molecular-weight heparin (enoxaparin) as prophylaxis against thromboembolism after total hip replacement. N Engl J Med 1996;335:696–700.
19 Planes A, Vocehlle N, Darmon J-Y, Fagola M, Bellaud M, Huet Y: Risk of deep-venous thrombosis after hospital discharge in patients having undergone total hip replacement: Double-blind randomised comparison of enoxaparin versus placebo. Lancet 1996;348:224–228.
20 Dahl OE, Andreassen G, Aspelin T, Muller C, Mathiesen P, Nyhus S, Abdelnoor M, Solhaug JH, Amesen H: Prolonged thromboprophylaxis following hip replacement surgery – results of a double-blind, prospective, randomised, placebo-controlled study with dalteparin (Fragmin). Thromb Haemost 1997;77:26–31.
21 Lassen MR, Borris LC, Anderson BS, Jensen HP, Skejo Bro HP, Andersen G, Petersen AO, Siem P, Horlyck E, Jensen BV, Thomsen PB, Hansen BR, Erin-Madsen J, Moller JC, Rotwitt L, Christensen F, Nielsen JB, Jorgensen PS, Paaske B, Torholm C, Hvidt P, Jensen NK, Nielsen AB, Appelquist E, Tjalve E: Efficacy and safety of prolonged thromboprophylaxis with a low molecular weight heparin (dalteparin) after total hip arthroplasty – the Danish Prolonged Prophylaxis (DaPP) Study. Thromb Res 1998; 89:281–287.
22 Hull RD, Brant RF, Pineo GF, Stein PD, Raskob GE, Valentine KA: Preoperative vs post-operative initiation of low-molecular-weight heparin prophylaxis against venous thromboembolism in patients undergoing elective hip replacement. Arch Intern Med 1999;159:137–141.
23 Pineo GF, Hull RD: A comparison of pre-operative dalteparin with post-operative dalteparin and with warfarin sodium for prophylaxis against DVT after total hip replacement during the acute hospital stay. Thromb Haemost 1999(suppl):Abstract 1194.
24 Hull RD, Raskob GE, Brant RF, Pineo GF: Subcutaneous low-molecular-weight heparin compared with continuous intravenous heparin in the treatment of patients with pulmonary embolism and underlying proximal deep-vein thrombosis. Thromb Haemost 1999(suppl):Abstract 19.
25 Clagget CP, Anderson FA, Geerts W, Heit JA, Knudson M, Lieberman JR, Merli G, Wheler HB: Prevention of venous thromboembolism. Chest 1998;114:531S–560S.

Main Paper

Hæmostasis

Haemostasis 1999;29(suppl 1):32–37

Low-Molecular-Weight Heparins in Coronary Thrombosis: Today and Tomorrow

L. Wallentin

Department of Cardiology, University Hospital, Uppsala, Sweden

Key Words
Low-molecular-weight heparins · Unstable coronary syndromes

Abstract
Data from several large-scale studies have suggested that low-molecular-weight heparin (LMWH) may be superior to standard heparin therapy in the setting of unstable coronary syndromes. Studies looking at the optimal duration of treatment have produced conflicting results; however, data from a recent large trial suggest that prolongation of treatment is associated with a significant benefit. The recommended initial treatment for patients with unstable coronary syndromes is a combination of LMWH and aspirin. Stablilized patients at moderate or high risk – such as those with ST-segment depression or increased troponin levels – should continue with this treatment until they have undergone coronary angiography and, if appropriate, an invasive procedure. In a recent small study among patients with acute myocardial infarction, the use of LMWH as an adjunct to streptokinase produced significant therapeutic benefits. Other potential uses for LMWH include a role in angioplasty.

Copyright © 1999 S. Karger AG, Basel

Introduction

All acute coronary syndromes share a common underlying pathophysiology. Rupture of an atherosclerotic plaque results in the formation of a thrombus, which impairs coronary blood flow and sometimes occludes the coronary artery. These coronary artery lesions are found in a spectrum of clinical syndromes, including unstable angina, where there is minor myocardial damage and elevation of biochemical markers. Data from a Swedish national registry regarding patients entering the coronary care unit (CCU) show that approximately a quarter of patients will have an acute myocardial infarction (MI). Around 10% will

KARGER

Fax + 41 61 306 12 34
E-Mail karger@karger.ch
www.karger.com

© 1999 S. Karger AG, Basel
0301–0147/99/0297–0032$17.50/0

Accessible online at:
www.karger.com/journals/hae

Prof. L. Wallentin
Department of Cardiology
University Hospital
S–751 23 Uppsala (Sweden)

have a diagnosis of unstable angina, and these patients, together with the 15% with a non-Q-wave MI, are considered to have an unstable coronary syndrome. Another 20% will be diagnosed as having stable angina, and some of these will also have a thrombus in their coronary artery, explaining the deterioration of their angina. Therefore, although there will be many other reasons for entering a CCU, around 55% of patients will have a coronary thrombus as an underlying pathophysiology.

Unstable coronary syndromes result from a combination of atherosclerotic, thrombotic and inflammatory processes. Patient categorization and risk stratification will help to determine the optimal treatment and identify patients whose risk of early progression is high. Although no single variable can be used alone, there is evidence to suggest that a number of biochemical markers, in combination with ECG findings, will provide valuable information. However, treatment strategies require improvement and further studies are needed to determine which patients should receive non-invasive management with antithrombotic medication and which require invasive procedures such as angioplasty or bypass surgery.

Risk Markers in Unstable Coronary Artery Disease (CAD)

Evidence from several sources demonstrates that the occurrence of ST episodes has implications for both the short-term and long-term outcome. In an interventional trial performed at the end of the 1980s, 800 patients were categorized according to their ECG at presentation: (1) chest pain without any ECG change; (2) T-wave inversions; (3) ST-segment depression, and (4) both ST-segment depression and elevation. The results showed that greater ST-segment changes were associated with an increased risk of MI [1]. In the FRISC (Fragmin During Instability in Coronary Artery Disease) II trial, 25–30% of the 200 participating patients had ST episodes and this group was at a considerably higher risk of death and/or MI over the study period of 3–6 months. These patients also had an increased need for revascularization [2]. Troponin is a well-established marker of myocardial damage and indicates poor prognosis in patients with chest pain and acute coronary syndromes [3, 4]. In the FRISC I trial, plasma levels of troponin T were determined at admission in 976 patients. The risk of death and MI over a 5-month period was considerably lower in the group with normal troponin levels. Patients with elevated levels had an almost four times greater risk of death and/or MI over the same time period [3]. Furthermore, the patients with elevated troponin levels showed a significant reduction in cardiac events during prolonged treatment with low-molecular-weight heparin (LMWH) [5]. Combining ECG and troponin observations provides additional information and further improves risk stratification [6]. Thus, patients with signs of ischaemia on the ECG and elevation of troponin levels are at considerably higher risk than are patients without these indicators [7].

The FRISC I trial also showed that signs of inflammatory activity can predict the risk of further cardiac events. Thus, increased levels of fibrinogen at presentation were independently associated with an increased risk of MI and/or mortality over the 5-month period of investigation. C-reactive protein (CRP) was also associated with increased mortality [8]. These results demonstrate that one in four patients with both elevated fibrinogen or CRP levels and increased troponin levels will have an MI or die within 5 months. Patients without any of these signs are at a significantly lower risk.

LMWH in Unstable CAD

Treatment of acute coronary syndromes should be related to the underlying pathophysiology. Rupture of a plaque exposes collagen, the lipid-rich core of the plaque and other thrombogenic substances, all of which stimulate the adhesion and aggregation of blood platelets. Platelet adhesion and aggregation can be attenuated with platelet inhibitors like aspirin, ADP inhibitors and glycoprotein (GP) IIb/IIIa inhibitors. Subsequent activation of the coagulation cascade converts soluble fibrinogen into insoluble fibrin. Strands of fibrin form a matrix of fibres that traps platelets and blood cells, resulting in the formation of a thrombus. This coagulation process can be attenuated with anticoagulants such as thrombin inhibitors, LMWH and standard heparin.

Several trials have demonstrated the efficacy of using either aspirin or heparin to treat unstable coronary disease. Subsequent trials have shown that the risk of MI and/or death is further reduced by using a combination of these two treatments [9]. However, discontinuation of heparin may be associated with reactivation of the disease process [10].

The use of LMWH avoids some of the disadvantages associated with standard heparin: poor subcutaneous bioavailability, dose-dependent clearance, variable anticoagulant effect, binding to phase-reactant proteins, and the need for laboratory monitoring [11].

The FRISC I trial was the first large-scale trial to demonstrate the efficacy of LMWH in patients with unstable coronary syndromes [12]. A total of 1,506 patients were treated with twice-daily doses of either dalteparin or placebo for the first 5–7 days. All patients also received aspirin. Treatment was subsequently continued with a once-daily dose of dalteparin or placebo. The trial demonstrated that dalteparin treatment resulted in a 63% relative reduction in the event rate, which was strongly significant, and in a 3.5% absolute reduction in death and MI maintained over 6 weeks.

Several trials have subsequently assessed standard heparin versus LMWH treatment in patients with unstable coronary syndromes. The FRIC (Fragmin in Unstable Coronary Artery Disease) trial, which randomized 1,498 patients to twice-daily dalteparin or standard heparin infusion for 5–7 days, demonstrated no differences in cardiac events between the two treatment groups [13]. Similarly, the Fraxiparin versus Unfractionated Heparin in Acute Coronary Syndromes (FRAX.I.S) trial in unstable CAD, which compared 2,317 patients randomized to at least 6 days of twice-daily subcutaneous nadroparin with 1,151 on heparin infusion for the same time period, demonstrated no differences in clinical outcome [14]. The ESSENCE (Efficacy and Safety of Subcutaneous Enoxaparin in Non-Q-Wave Coronary Events) trial included 3,171 patients who received enoxaparin or heparin for 2–8 days in addition to aspirin therapy [15]. In this comparison, enoxaparin was significantly more effective in reducing the incidence of the composite endpoint (death, MI or recurrent angina) at both 14 and 30 days. This result was recently confirmed in the preliminary reported and similar TIMI (Thrombolysis in Myocardial Infarction) 11B trial, which compared enoxaparin for a median time of 4.5 days with heparin infusion for a median of 3 days [16].

Although antithrombotic treatment is normally given for less than a week, there is a rationale for more prolonged treatment. A thrombus at a coronary lesion lasts for several months and coagulation activity is elevated for at least 3 months [17, 18]. Furthermore, the long-term results of the FRISC I trial demonstrated that lowering the dose or termination of treatment too early results in the loss of some of the treatment benefit [12].

Several trials have recently studied short-term versus long-term treatment in unstable CAD. In the TIMI 11B trial [16], patients received twice-daily treatment with enoxaparin or standard heparin until either hospital discharge or day 8. Thereafter they continued on either a standard twice-daily dose of 40–60 mg enoxaparin or placebo for a further 40 days. The composite endpoint (death, MI or revascularization) was significantly lower with enoxaparin than with standard heparin at 14 days, and this benefit was sustained with prolonged treatment. The FRAX.I.S trial showed no advantage of continuation with twice-daily nadroparin for 14 days compared with either nadroparin or unfractionated heparin treatment for 6 ± 2 days [14]. The FRIC trial included 1,482 patients and demonstrated no difference in outcome during prolonged (days 6–45) treatment with once-daily dalteparin in comparison with placebo [13]. In the FRISC II medical trial, all patients received aspirin and dalteparin for 5–7 days and were subsequently randomized to receive twice-daily dalteparin or placebo for up to 3 months [19]. In contrast with the other trials, in the non-invasively managed cohort, the FRISC II study showed a significant benefit of the prolonged treatment, with a 30–40% reduction in death and MI during the first 2 months and a significant decrease in the composite endpoint of death, MI and revascularization lasting for the whole treatment period [20].

Revascularization in Unstable CAD

Unstable coronary syndromes can be treated using either an early invasive approach or a non-invasive approach. With the former, patients undergo a coronary angiogram and, if appropriate, revascularization within a few days; with the latter, only patients with severe ischaemia or refractory symptoms are referred for revascularization. The two strategies were compared in the FRISC II trial, which randomized 1,222 patients to coronary angiography and invasive procedures within 1 week (either percutaneous coronary intervention or coronary artery bypass surgery, depending on the individual patient) and 1,235 patients to a non-invasive approach. Although the patients undergoing invasive procedures had an increased initial risk of procedure-related MI, after 6 months the invasive strategy was associated with a significant 22% relative reduction in death and MI, which also corresponded to a reduction in total mortality [21].

Treatment Recommendations in Unstable CAD

Based on the results obtained, the recommended initial treatment for patients with unstable coronary syndromes is a combination of LMWH and aspirin. If, despite this regimen, patients have signs of severe ischaemia, the addition of a GPIIb/IIIa blocker and urgent revascularization should be considered. The follow-on strategy used in stabilized patients at moderate or high risk should be continuation with aspirin and LMWH until the patient has undergone coronary angiography and, if appropriate, an invasive procedure. The lowest-risk patients will, after the initial phase, require only aspirin and antianginal drugs, without further anticoagulant drugs and without any need for revascularization [22].

LMWH in Acute ST-Elevation MI

Patients with total occlusion and ST elevation usually undergo early reperfusion; however, this is often incomplete and TIMI 3 flow (full flow at 90 min) is obtained in only approximately 50–60% of patients. Both standard-dose and accelerated tissue plasminogen activator have an inadequate thrombolytic effect and there are problems achieving early patency [23]. The rebound phenomenon occurs when heparin treatment is stopped, and this results in an increased number of events. There is also inadequate inhibition of the platelets activated by both MI and thrombolytic treatment. Studies have suggested that LMWH might be useful as an adjuvant to thrombolytics in this setting. In the recent BIOMACS (Biochemical Markers in Acute Coronary Syndromes) trial, 101 patients with acute MI were randomized to two injections of dalteparin or placebo, one just before streptokinase and the other 12 h later [24]. The effects were evaluated by coronary angiograms after 20–28 h, and the influence of treatment on non-invasive markers of early reperfusion and recurrent ischaemia were also assessed. The TIMI 3 blood flow increased by 15–20% in patients receiving dalteparin, and this improvement was significant in patients with non-invasive signs of reperfusion at 90 min. There was also a reduction in episodes of ischaemia in the dalteparin-treated group, indicating that treatment resulted in more stable coronary blood flow and less thrombus formation after thrombolysis. The study also demonstrated a reduction in coagulation activity in the treated patients, which might be related to the improved coronary blood flow. Although this study was small, the results indicated that adding LMWH to fibrinolytics in patients with ST-segment elevation might produce substantial benefits. There are now several ongoing trials using LMWH in thrombolysed patients and it is hoped that these trials will improve early reperfusion and result in a better patency.

Future of LMWH in Coronary Thrombosis

LMWHs may be routinely used in patients with unstable coronary syndromes. They may eventually also replace standard heparin as an adjuvant to fibrinolytic agents, because, together with an intravenous bolus of a thrombolytic agent, they constitute the ideal treatment in the prehospital setting. LMWH might also replace standard heparin in angioplasty; several trials have shown that, although LMWHs do not reduce the rate of restenosis, they offer a safe alternative to intravenous heparin at angioplasty procedures. Because LMWHs are replacing standard heparin in many conditions with coronary thrombi, their efficacy and safety when used in combination with new platelet inhibitors – i.e. ADP inhibitors and GPIIb/IIIa inhibitors – needs to be evaluated. Based on current knowledge, LMWHs seem to have become a replacement for standard heparin in all manifestations of acute coronary thrombosis.

References

1 Nyman I, Areskog M, Areskog NH, Swahn E, Wallentin L, for the RISC Study Group: Very early risk stratification by electrocardiogram at rest in men with suspected unstable coronary heart disease. J Intern Med 1993;234:293–301.

2 Jernberg T, Lindahl B, Chronblad J, Wallentin L: ST-segment monitoring with continuous 12-lead ECG identifies patients at high risk for subsequent cardiac events after an episode of unstable coronary artery disease (abstract). European Congress Cardiology 1999.

3 Lindahl B, Venge P, Wallentin L, for the FRISC Study Group: Relation between troponin T and the risk of subsequent cardiac events in unstable coronary artery disease. Circulation 1996;93:1651–1657.

4 Ohman EM, Armstrong PW, Christenson RH, Granger CB, Katus HA, Hamm CW, O'Hanesian MA, Wagner GS, Kleiman NS, Harrell FE Jr, Califf RM, Topol EJ: Cardiac troponin T levels for risk stratification in acute myocardial ischemia. N Engl J Med 1996;335:1333–1341.
5 Lindahl B, Venge P, Wallentin L: Troponin T identifies patients with unstable coronary artery disease who benefit from long-term antithrombotic protection. J Am Coll Cardiol 1997;29:43–48.
6 Holmvang L, Luscher MS, Clemmensen P, Thygesen K, Grande P, for the TRIM Study Group: Very early risk stratification using combined ECG and biochemical assessment in patients with unstable coronary artery disease [A Thrombin Inhibition in Myocardial Ischemia (TRIM) substudy]. Circulation 1998;98:2004–2009.
7 Norgaard BL, Andersen K, Dellborg M, Abrahamsson P, Ravkilde J, Thygesen K, for the TRIM (Thrombin Inhibition in Myocardial Ischaemia) Study Group: Admission risk assessment by cardiac troponin T in unstable coronary artery disease: Additional prognostic information from continuous ST segment monitoring. J Am Coll Cardiol 1999;33:1519–1527.
8 Toss H, Lindahl B, Siegbahn A, Wallentin L, for the FRISC (Fragmin During Instability in Coronary Artery Disease) Study Group: Prognostic influence of increased fibrinogen and C-reactive protein levels in unstable coronary artery disease. Circulation 1997;96:4204–4210.
9 Oler A, Whooley MA, Oler J, Grady D: Adding heparin to aspirin reduces the incidence of myocardial infarction and death in patients with unstable angina. A meta-analysis. J Am Med Assoc 1996;276:811–815.
10 Theroux P, Waters D, Lam J, Juneau M, McCans J: Reactivation of unstable angina after the discontinuation of heparin. N Engl J Med 1992;327:141–145.
11 Hirsh J, Dalen JE, Deykin D, Poller L: Heparin: Mechanism of action, pharmacokinetics, dosing considerations, monitoring, efficacy, and safety. Chest 1992;102(suppl 4):337S–351S.
12 Fragmin During Instability in Coronary Artery Disease (FRISC) Study Group: Low-molecular-weight heparin during instability in coronary artery disease. Lancet 1996;347:561–568.
13 Klein W, Buchwald A, Hillis SE, Monrad S, Sanz G, Turpie AGG, van der Meer J, Olaisson E, Undeland S, Lundwig K: Comparison of low-molecular-weight heparin with unfractionated heparin acutely and with placebo for 6 weeks in the management of unstable coronary artery disease. Circulation 1997;96:61–68.
14 Leizorovicz A, for the FRAX.I.S group: Comparison of two treatment durations (6 and 14 days) of a low molecular weight heparin with a 6 day treatment of unfractionated heparin in the initial management of unstable angina or non-Q-wave myocardial infarction. Eur Heart J 1999, in press.
15 Cohen M, Demers C, Gurfinkel EP, Turpie AGG, Fromell GJ, Goodman S, Langer A, Califf RM, Fox KAA, Premmereur J, Bigonzi F: A comparison of low-molecular-weight heparin with unfractionated heparin for unstable coronary artery disease. N Engl J Med 1997;337:447–452.
16 Antman EM, for the Thrombolysis in Myocardial Infarction (TIMI) 11B Investigators: Enoxaparin versus unfractionated heparin for unstable angina or non-Q-wave myocardial infarction: A double-blind, placebo-controlled, parallel-group, multicenter trial. Rationale, study design, and methods. Am Heart J 1998;135(6 Pt 3 suppl):S353–S360.
17 Van Belle E, Lablanche JM, Bauters C, Renaud N, McFadden EP, Bertrand ME: Coronary angioscopic findings in the infarct-related vessel within 1 month of acute myocardial infarction: Natural history and the effect of thrombolysis. Circulation 1998;97:26–33.
18 Merlini PA, Bauer KA, Oltrona L, Ardissino D, Cattaneo M, Belli C, Mannucci PM, Rosenberg, RD: Persistent activation of coagulation mechanism in unstable angina and myocardial infarction. Circulation 1994;90:61–68.
19 Wallentin L, Husted S, Kontny F, Swahn E: Long-term low-molecular-weight heparin (Fragmin) and/or early revascularization during instability in coronary artery disease (the FRISC II study). Am J Cardiol 1997;80:61E–63E.
20 The Fragmin During Instability in Coronary Artery Disease (FRISC II) Investigators: Long-term low molecular mass heparin (dalteparin) in unstable coronary artery disease – a prospective randomised multicentre study – the FRISC II medical trial. Lancet 1999;354:701–707.
21 The Fragmin During Instability in Coronary Artery Disease (FRISC II) Investigators: Invasive versus non-invasive strategy in unstable coronary artery disease – a prospective randomised multicentre study – the FRISC II invasive trial. Lancet 1999;354:708–715.
22 Campbell RW, Wallentin L, Verheugt FW, Turpie AG, Maseri A, Klein W, Cleland JG, Bode C, Becker R, Anderson J, Bertrand ME, Conti CR: Management strategies for a better outcome in unstable coronary artery disease. Clin Cardiol 1998;21:314–322.
23 Barbagelata NA, Granger CB, Oqueli E, Suarez LD, Borruel M, Topol EJ, Califf RM: TIMI grade 3 flow and reocclusion after intravenous thrombolytic therapy: A pooled analysis. Am Heart J 1997;133:273–282.
24 Frostfeldt G, Ahlberg G, Gustafsson G, Helmius G, Lindahl B, Nygren A, Siegbahn A, Swahn E, Venge P, Wallentin L: Low molecular weight heparin (dalteparin) as adjuvant treatment of thrombolysis in acute myocardial infarction – a pilot study: Biochemical markers in acute coronary syndromes (BIOMACS II). J Am Coll Cardiol 1999;33:627–633.

Main Paper

Hæmostasis

Haemostasis 1999;29(suppl 1):38–47

What Else Can 'Heparin' Do?

Ulf Lindahl

Department of Medical Biochemistry and Microbiology, The Biomedical Centre, University of Uppsala, Uppsala, Sweden

Key Words

Growth factors · Heparin · Heparan sulphate · *L*-iduronic acid · Protein binding · Sulphation

Abstract

This review article begins by discussing the molecular basis of the blood anticoagulant effect of heparin and some species of heparan sulphate (HS). A highly specific pentasaccharide sequence, containing a glucosamine 3-O-sulphate group, is a key structural element for this action. The biosynthesis of heparin and HS is outlined. Different types of HS proteoglycans exist. Analysis of HS preparations from different mammalian organs has indicated that the structural variability of the polysaccharide is due to regulated polymer modification. In addition to antithrombin, HS chains bind a very large number of other proteins in vivo. Such binding often appears to depend on the presence of specific sequences of different monosaccharide building-blocks and has diverse implications. Many physiological and pathological processes in the mammalian body appear to be influenced or regulated by HS proteoglycans. For example, the proper assembly of HS chains is believed to play an important role in normal embryonic and mammalian development. Diseases such as diabetes, amyloidosis and Alzheimer's may be associated with changes in HS structure. Finally, the possibilities and strategies for developing drugs based on HS chemistry are discussed.

Copyright © 1999 S. Karger AG, Basel

Heparin Prevents Blood Coagulation ...

The blood anticoagulant effect of heparin, a glycosaminoglycan, is widely exploited in the clinic to prevent and treat thromboembolic disease. The molecular basis of this effect has been investigated in detail [1, 2]. A pentasaccharide domain of the polysaccharide chain binds to antithrombin (AT), and

KARGER

Fax + 41 61 306 12 34
E-Mail karger@karger.ch
www.karger.com

© 1999 S. Karger AG, Basel
0301–0147/99/0297–0038$17.50/0

Accessible online at:
www.karger.com/journals/hae

Dr. U. Lindahl
Department of Medical Biochemistry and Microbiology
The Biomedical Centre
University of Uppsala, Box 575
S–751 23 Uppsala (Sweden)

thus greatly accelerates the rate at which this proteinase inhibitor inactivates thrombin and other coagulation enzymes (fig. 1A). The structure of the pentasaccharide sequence is highly specific, and is distinguished in particular by the occurrence of a glucosamine 3-O-sulphate group that is only rarely seen in other regions of the polymer. The pentasaccharide sequence is a key structural element also in low-molecular-weight heparin (LMWH), a heparin derivative of Mr ~ 5,000 that has been trimmed down to about one-third the size of the original chain. This product thus binds avidly to AT but is just barely able also to bind thrombin adjacent to the AT-binding site, apparently a prerequisite for antithrombotic action [2] (fig. 1B). Truncation of the further extended saccharide sequences eliminates interactions between the heparin chain and a multitude of other proteins, and thereby induces the favourable pharmacokinetic and dosage properties of the drug.

... And So Do Some Species of Heparan Sulphate (HS)

Heparin is synthesized and stored, as serglycin proteoglycans, in connective-tissue-type mast cells [3]. The functional role of this macromolecule is unclear; a function in the regulation of blood coagulation appears unlikely. Instead, HS proteoglycans, located on vascular endothelial surfaces, express the AT-binding pentasaccharide sequence, and are capable of potentiating the inactivation of coagulation enzymes [4].

The HS proteoglycans are of different types [5, 6]. Two major families of such species are the syndecans and glypicans, both of which have several members and occur at cell surfaces. The syndecan core proteins are intercalated in cell membranes, whereas the glypicans are attached through phosphatidylinositol anchors. The major extracellular HS proteoglycans are perlecan and agrin.

A Selective Modulator of Protein Functions

In addition to AT, heparin binds a very large number of other proteins, including enzymes, enzyme inhibitors, growth factors and chemokines, extracellular matrix components, cell adhesion molecules and microbial proteins. The interactions are largely electrostatic, owing to the polyanionic nature of the polysaccharide, and because so many different proteins apparently bind to the same polyanion sequence, the interactions are generally held to be 'non-specific'. However, most of these proteins presumably bind to HS rather than to heparin chains in vivo, thus potentially implicating HS in a variety of processes of physiological or pathophysiological importance (table 1). Indeed, minimal structural requirements for binding, expressed by a given HS species in relation to a defined protein ligand, may be obscured in heparin due to redundant sulphation [7]. This concept is best understood through a brief account of heparin and HS biosynthesis.

The biosynthetic process involves the initial formation of a [*D*-glucuronic acid – *N*-acetyl-*D*-glucosamine]$_n$ ([GlcA-GlcNAc]$_n$) poly-

Table 1. Potential/proposed roles for HS in vivo

Modulation of growth factor action (embryonic development)
Inhibition of blood coagulation
Anchorage of cells
Organization of extracellular matrix
Angiogenesis
Positioning of enzymes and cytokines at cell surfaces
'Co-receptor' function in viral infections

mer that is subsequently modified by partial N-deacetylation/N-sulphation of GlcNAc units, C5-epimerization (inversion of configuration at carbon 5) of GlcA to *L*-iduronic acid (IdoA) units, and, finally, incorporation of O-sulphate groups at different positions [8]. Polymer modification occurs in a sequential manner, such that the products of previous reactions will provide substrate residues for subsequent steps, and is clearly constrained by the substrate specificities of the various enzymes that catalyse these steps. The C5-epimerization and O-sulphation reactions thus depend on the previous incorporation of N-sulphate groups, and therefore tend to generate domains of more or less extensively modified saccharide sequences. Heparin (fig. 2A) is heavily N- and O-sulphated, and thus more homogenous than HS chains (fig. 2B), which are generally irregular in structure and show marked domain organization. Even within the N-sulphated domains, the HS chains are only partially epimerized and O-sulphated, giving rise to extensive sequence heterogeneity. The mechanisms in control of this variability remain poorly understood but appear to depend on the involvement of distinct enzyme isoforms with different substrate-recognition properties [8]. Comparing the (hypothetical) sequences of the biosynthetic products in figures 2A and B, it is readily appreciated that proteins that bind in a selective manner to different HS sequences may all interact with the same heparin chain.

Analysis of HS preparations from different mammalian organs strongly supports the notion that the structural variability of the polysaccharide is due to regulated rather than random polymer modification [9–11]. Moreover, immunohistochemical staining of rat kidney sections with monoclonal antibodies that recognize different HS epitopes revealed distinct staining patterns that could only be explained by the occurrence of different HS species with distinct topology in relation to different cell types [12, 13]. We assume that these patterns reflect the requirements for distinct HS structures in interactions with various proteins.

The protein-binding HS sequences investigated so far seem generally not to depend on the presence of 'unique' components (such as the 3-O-sulphate group in the AT-binding pentasaccharide sequence), inasmuch as they are composed of the commonly occurring major HS building-blocks. Notably, such an arrangement does not exclude selectivity in binding. Binding of basic fibroblast growth factor (FGF-2) thus requires an N-sulphated HS pentamer sequence containing a single

Fig. 1. A Schematic outline of the anticoagulant action of heparin, including the structure of the pentasaccharide sequence required to bind, immobilize and activate AT. **B** Principal structural difference between conventional heparin and low-molecular-weight heparin (LMWH). Both sequences display the specific AT-binding pentasaccharide sequence. Most of the additional saccharide sequences of the native heparin chain have been removed to generate LMWH, thus minimizing interactions with proteins other than AT. The structure of the pentasaccharide sequence is highly specific, and is distinguished in particular by the occurrence of a glucosamine 3-O-sulphate group that is only rarely seen in other regions of the polymer. The pentasaccharide sequence is a key structural element also in LMWH, a heparin derivative of Mr ~ 5,000 that has been trimmed down to about one-third the size of the original chain. This product thus binds avidly to AT but is just barely able also to bind thrombin adjacent to the AT-binding site, apparently a prerequisite for antithrombotic action.

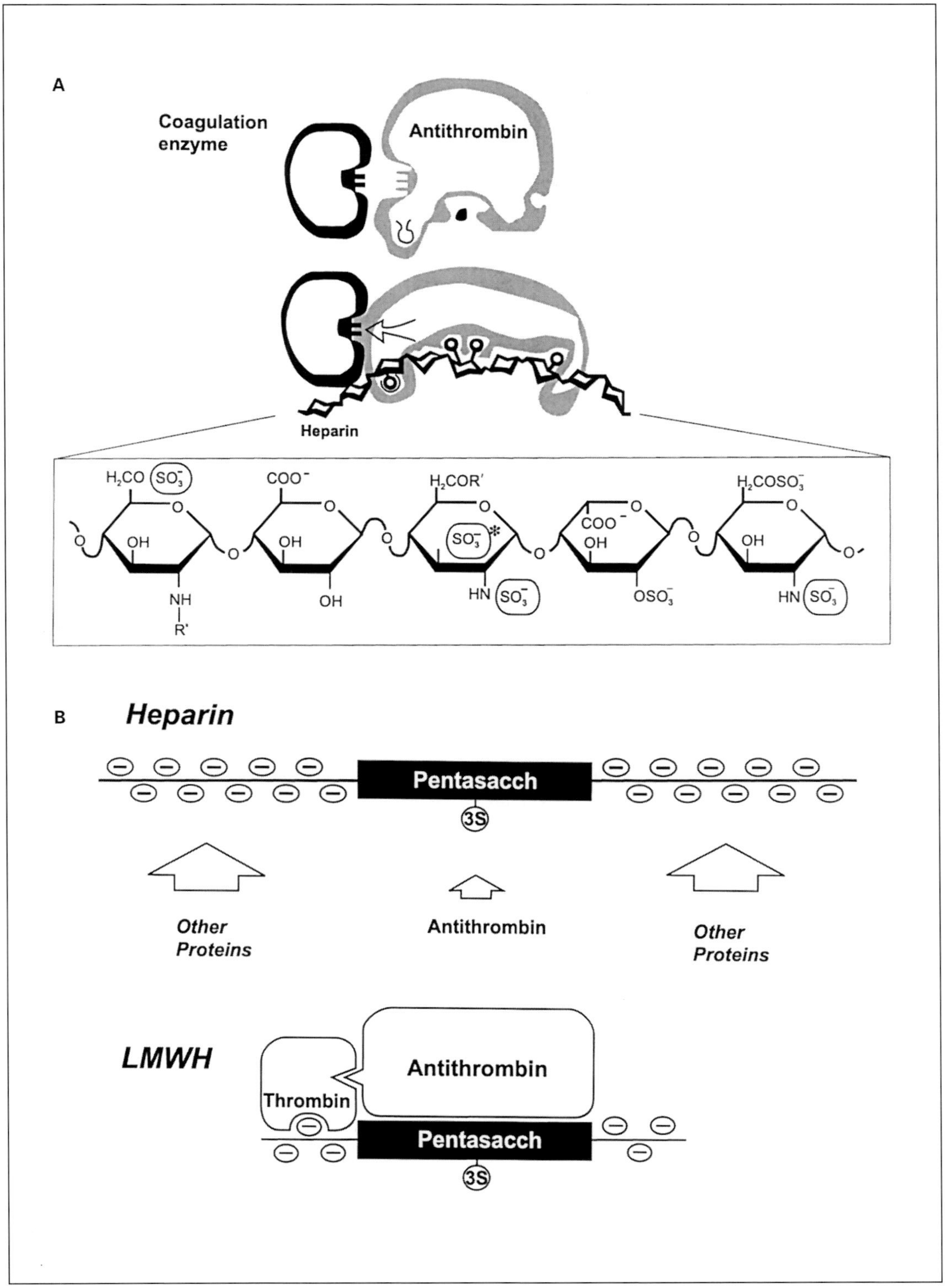
A
Coagulation enzyme
Antithrombin
Heparin
B
Heparin
Pentasacch
3S
Other Proteins
Antithrombin
Other Proteins
LMWH
Thrombin
Antithrombin
Pentasacch
3S

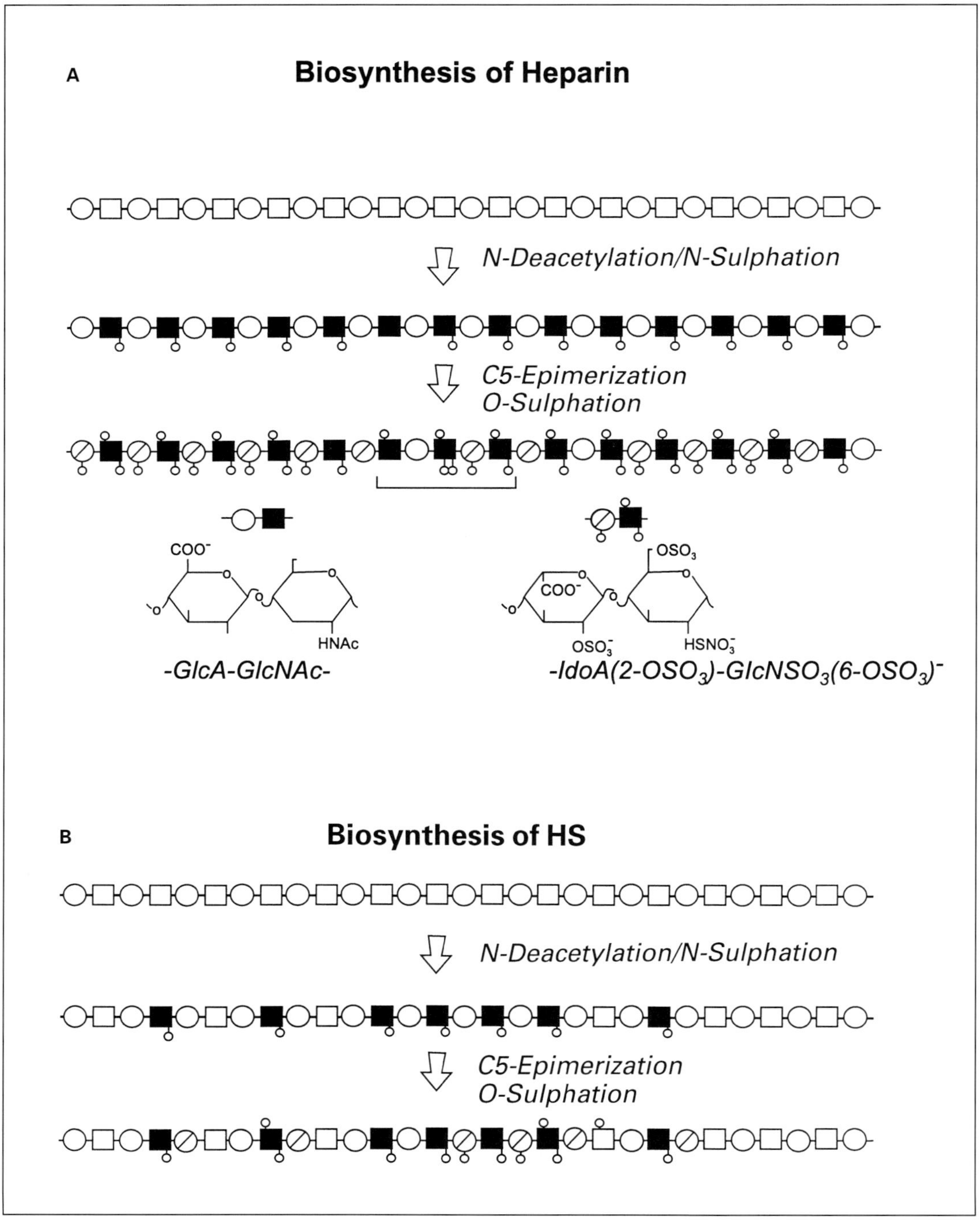

Fig. 2. Schematics illustrating the polymer-modification reactions involved in the biosynthesis of heparin (**A**) and HS (**B**). The chemical structures corresponding to the various symbols are defined through the disaccharides shown in detail under the scheme in panel A. The bracket in panel A indicates the AT-binding pentasaccharide sequence.

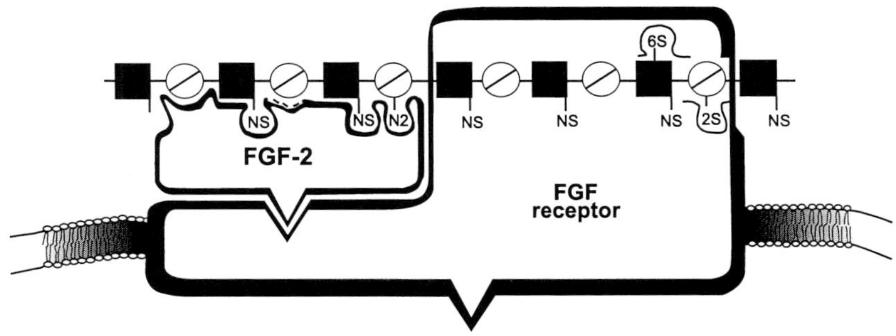

Fig. 3. Hypothetical model of the proposed ternary complex involving HS, FGF-2 and the FGF receptor. The model indicates in tentative fashion (no direct sequence information yet available) that different saccharide structures in the HS chain are required for interactions with the growth factor molecule and with its receptor.

IdoA 2-O-sulphate group but no GlcN 6-O-sulphate residues; the latter substituents are tolerated but are not essential for binding [14, 15]. On the other hand, interactions with several other proteins, including lipoprotein lipase [16], hepatocyte growth factor [17], platelet-derived growth factor (PDGF) [18] and herpes simplex gC glycoprotein [19] all depend on the occurrence of at least one GlcN 6-O-sulphate group. This requirement was generally demonstrated through the preferential binding of oligosaccharides containing the trisulphated disaccharide unit IdoA(2-OSO_3)-GlcNSO_3(6-OSO_3). This particular disaccharide unit, abundant in heparin chains but highly variable in HS species (fig. 2), is formed by 6-O-sulphation, presumably tightly regulated, of previously 2-O-sulphated saccharide sequences.

The functional implications of protein binding to HS chains are diverse. The HS-bound proteins (e.g. PDGF) may simply be sequestered at the cell surface, or in the extracellular matrix, protected against proteolytic degradation, until they are mobilized by partial cleavage of the HS carrier by a specific heparanase [20]. Chemokines may be positioned, via an HS chain, for interaction with their receptors on other cells [21, 22]. Interactions between proteins (e.g. *L*-selectin) and subsets of HS proteoglycans may directly contribute to various cell adhesion phenomena [23]. Finally, such interactions may be directly required for expression of a particular biological activity. It thus is now apparent that many growth factors require binding to HS chains at the cell surface, as first proposed for FGF-2 [24], in order to promote cell proliferation. More detailed analysis suggested that productive association of FGF-2 with its receptor involves two adjacent but structurally different ~ 6-mer HS domains [25, 26], conceivably designed for simultaneous binding of the growth factor and receptor molecules [27] (fig. 3). Future research will undoubtedly reveal equally elaborate interactions with distinct HS structures behind the functions of many different proteins.

In Development, Health and Disease

Genetic screens in *Drosophila* have identified several genes of fundamental importance for normal embryonic development. More recent molecular-genetic analysis of HS proteoglycans and their biosynthesis revealed that some of these essential genes encode core proteins for HS proteoglycans or biosynthetic enzymes required for the proper assembly of HS chains [28]. Such enzymes have been implicated also in mammalian development. For example, loss of the enzyme that catalyses 2-O-sulphation of IdoA units in HS leads to severe malformations in the rat, including absence of kidneys [29]. More subtle phenotype modulations have been observed also. Targeted disruption of one of the N-deacetylase/N-sulphotransferase isoforms involved in the initial polymer-modification reaction (fig. 2) thus led to the formation of abnormal connective-tissue-type mast cells, unable to produce heparin, in otherwise seemingly healthy mice [30]. Further, development/aging has been associated with changes in HS composition. For example, development of the embryonic rat brain entails a distinct switch in HS-mediated growth factor activity between members of the FGF family, from FGF-2 to FGF-1 [31]. This transition, which occurs along with a change from proliferation of neural precursor cells to neuronal differentiation, is accompanied by subtle structural modulation of the predominant HS species involving, in particular, the pattern of 6-O-sulphation. Moreover, an age-related increase in GlcN 6-O-sulphation of human aortic HS was accompanied by dramatically increased binding of PDGF isoforms [32] and of FGF-1 [33] but not of FGF-2 [32, 33]. Intriguing functional roles have been ascribed to syndecan-attached HS at the surface of neuronal cells in the rat brain. The interaction between this HS species and brain-specific HS-binding proteins – in particular, heparin-binding growth-associated molecule (HB-GAM) – has been implicated in the control of neurite outgrowth [34], as well as in the induction of synaptic long-term potentiation, believed to be essential for the evolvement of memory [35].

Although changes in the sulphation pattern of HS in response to 'differentiation' or 'transformation' of cells in culture have been reported [see, for example, 36, 37 and references therein], consistent changes in HS structure associated with tumours have not been described. Other diseases may be associated with changes in HS structure. Experimentally induced diabetes in rats thus resulted in decreased N-sulphation of hepatic HS [38] [for further reading, please see Van der Woude's paper, p. 61]. Moreover, analysis of HS accumulated in internal organs of patients with amyloid-A amyloidosis revealed a switch in O-sulphation, to a novel pattern that was common to the amyloid-associated HS from different organs but differed from the distinct sulphation profiles characteristic for the HS species of the corresponding normal organs (liver and spleen) [39]. In Alzheimer's disease, another amyloidotic condition, HS has been directly implicated in the generation of the typical lesions, neuritic plaques [40, 41] and paired helical filaments [42]. Moreover, an HS proteoglycan appears to serve as a coreceptor for Aβ fibrils as they activate microglia to produce neurotoxic agents and induce neurone death [43].

Drugs Based on HS Chemistry?

The multitude of physiological and pathological processes in the mammalian body that appear to be influenced/regulated by HS proteoglycans raises the prospect of drug development based on HS chemistry. Clearly, such pursuit must be guided by aspects of specifici-

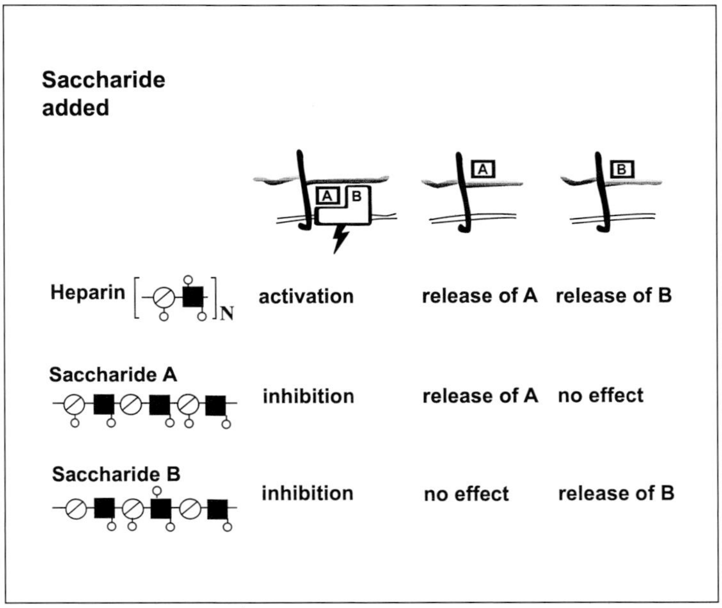

Fig. 4. Predicted effects of added saccharides on interactions between cell-surface HS proteoglycans and protein ligands. If the function of the endogenous HS proteoglycan is simply to immobilize the protein ligand (e.g. a chemokine in an inflammatory condition), the effects of added saccharides are readily predicted. Heparin would displace both proteins, whereas saccharides A and B would be selective.

ty and selectivity in the interactions of HS with proteins, as outlined above. Conversely, we are intrigued by the potential number of such interactions in the patient that are unintentionally disrupted in the course of conventional heparin therapy. For example, it was calculated that P- and *L*-selectin binding to sialyl-Lewis$_x$ and to HL-60 cells is inhibited by unfractionated pharmaceutical heparin preparations at concentrations 12- to 50-fold lower than those recommended for effective anticoagulation in vivo. Interestingly, LMWH preparations appear to be much poorer inhibitors [44].

An attempt to highlight these differences is given in figure 4. Two distinct (hypothetical) saccharide epitopes, designated A and B, are assumed to interact with their cognate proteins. Assuming that these epitopes are expressed by different HS species, but are both mimicked (albeit in 'masked' form; see above) by heparin, the predicted effects of added (non-selective) heparin or (selective) HS species vary depending on the functional context. If the two proteins represent a growth factor and its cell-surface receptor, heparin would potentially promote receptor activation (similar to an HS chain containing both A and B epitopes), whereas either one of the HS species would be inhibitory (due to blocking of either the growth factor or the receptor). Notably, drugs may be required that either stimulate (e.g. wound healing) or inhibit (e.g. angiogenesis in cancer treatment) the action of 'heparin-dependent' growth factors, such as FGF-2. If the function of the endogenous HS proteoglycan is simply to immobilize the protein ligand (e.g. a chemokine in an inflammatory condition), the effects of added saccharides are readily predicted. Heparin would displace both proteins, whereas saccharides A and B would be selective (fig. 4). The strategies for developing drugs with selective action would primarily be based on detailed assessment at the atomic level of the appropriate saccharide–protein interactions, with special emphasis on the precise location of essential charged groups (such as sulphate residues). Further development would involve either chemical synthesis of a saccharide with optimal structure, or the generation of a simplified 'glycomimetic', not necessarily containing sugar residues, that expresses the particular molecular features required for protein interaction [2]. The possibilities offered by such strategies clearly deserve more attention than they have so far received.

References

1 Bourin M-C, Lindahl U: Glycosaminoglycans and the regulation of blood coagulation. Biochem J 1993; 289:313–330.
2 Petitou M, Herault JP, Driguez PA, Duchaussoy P, Lormeau, JC, Herbert JM: Synthesis of thrombin-inhibiting heparin mimetics without side effects. Nature 1999;398:417–422.
3 Lidholt K, Eriksson I, Kjellén L: Heparin proteoglycans synthesized by mouse mastocytoma contain chondroitin sulfate. Biochem J 1995:311:233–238.
4 Rosenberg RD, Shworak NW, Liu J, Schwartz JJ, Zhang L: Heparan sulfate proteoglycans of the cardiovascular system. Specific structures emerge but how is synthesis regulated? J Clin Invest 1997;100(suppl 11):S67–S75.
5 David G: Integral membrane heparan sulfate proteoglycans. FASEB Journal 1993;7:1023–1030.
6 Iozzo RV: Matrix proteoglycans: From molecular design to cellular function. Ann Rev Biochem 1998; 67:609–652.
7 Salmivirta M, Lidholt K, Lindahl U: Heparan sulfate – a piece of information. FASEB Journal 1996;10: 1270–1279.
8 Lindahl U, Kusche-Gullberg M, Kjellen L: Regulated diversity of heparan sulfate. J Biol Chem 1998; 273:24979–24982.
9 Lyon M, Deakin JA, Gallagher JT: Liver heparan sulfate structure. A novel molecular design. J Biol Chem 1994;269:11208–11215.
10 Lindahl B, Eriksson L, Lindahl U: Structure of heparan sulfate from human brain, with special regard to Alzheimer's disease. Biochem J 1995;306:177–184.
11 Maccarana M, Sakura Y, Tawada A, Yoshida K, Lindahl U: Domain structure of heparan sulfates from bovine organs. J Biol Chem 1996; 271:17804–17810.
12 van den Born J, Gunnarsson K, Bakker MA, Kjellen L, Kusche-Gullberg M, Maccarana M, Berden JH, Lindahl U: Presence of N-unsubstituted glucosamine units in native heparan sulfate revealed by a monoclonal antibody. J Biol Chem 1995;270:31303–31309.
13 van Kuppevelt TH, Dennissen MA, van Venrooij WJ, Hoet RM, Veerkamp JH: Generation and application of type-specific anti-heparan sulfate antibodies using phage display technology. Further evidence for heparan sulfate heterogeneity in the kidney. J Biol Chem 1998;273: 12960–12966.
14 Maccarana M, Casu B, Lindahl U: Minimal sequence in heparin/heparan sulfate required for binding of basic fibroblast growth factor. J Biol Chem 1993;268:23898–23905.
15 Faham S, Hileman RE, Fromm JR, Linhardt RJ, Rees DC: Heparin structure and interactions with basic fibroblast growth factors. Science 1996;271:1116–1120.
16 Parthasarathy N, Goldberg IJ, Sivarau P, Mulloy B, Flory DM, Wagner WD: Oligosaccharide sequences of endothelial cell surface heparan sulfate proteoglycan with affinity for lipoprotein lipase. J Biol Chem 1994;269:22391–22396.
17 Lyon M, Deakin JA, Mizuno K, Nakamura T, Gallagher JT: Interaction of hepatocyte growth factor with heparan sulfate. J Biol Chem 1994; 269:11216–11223.
18 Feyzi E, Lustig F, Fager G, Spillmann D, Lindahl U, Salmivirta M: Characterization of heparin and heparan sulfate domains binding to the long splice variant of platelet-derived growth factor A chain. J Biol Chem 1997;272:5518–5524.
19 Feyzi E, Trybala E, Bergstrom T, Lindahl U, Spillmann D: Structural requirement of heparan sulfate for interaction with Herpes simplex virus type 1 virions and isolated glycoprotein C. J Biol Chem 1997;272: 24850–24857.
20 Vlodavsky I, Bar-Shavit R, Ishai-Michaeli R, Bashkin P, Fuks Z: Extracellular sequestration and release of fibroblast growth factor: A regulatory mechanism? Trends Biochem Sci 1991;16:268–271.
21 Tanaka Y, Adams DH, Huscher S, Hirano H, Siebenlist U, Shaw S: T-cell adhesion induced by proteoglycan-immobilized cytokine MIP–1βετα. Nature 1993;361:79–82.
22 Spillmann D, Witt D, Lindahl U: Defining the interleukin-8-binding domain of heparan sulfate. J Biol Chem 1998;273:15487–15493.
23 Norgard-Sumnicht K, Varki A: Endothelial heparan sulfate proteoglycans that bind to *L*-selectin have glucosamine residues with unsubstituted amino groups. J Biol Chem 1995;270:12012–12024.
24 Rapraeger AC, Krufka A, Olwin BB: Requirement of heparan sulfate for bFGF-mediated fibroblast growth and myoblast differentiation. Science 1991;252:1705–1708.
25 Guimond S, Maccarana M, Olwin BB, Lindahl U, Rapraeger AC: Activating and inhibitory heparin sequences for FGF-2 (basic FGF). Distinct requirements for FGF-1, FGF-2, and FGF-4. J Biol Chem 1993;268:23906–23914.

26 Pye DA, Vives RR, Turnbull JE, Hyde P, Gallagher JT: Heparan sulfate oligosaccharides require 6-O-sulfation for promotion of basic fibroblast growth factor mitogenic activity. J Biol Chem 1998;273:22936–22942.
27 Pantoliano MW, Springer BA, Van Dyk DE, Tobery T, Wetmore DR, Lear JD, Nahapetian AT, Bradley JD, Sisk WP: Multivalent ligand-receptor binding interactions in the fibroblast growth factor system produce a cooperative growth factor and heparin mechanism for receptor dimerization. Biochemistry 1994;33:10229–10248.
28 Selleck S: Genetic analysis of functions for cell surface proteoglycans. Matrix Biol 1998;17:473–476.
29 Bullock SL, Fletcher JM, Beddington RS, Wilson VA: Renal agenesis in mice homozygous for a gene trap mutation in the gene encoding heparan sulfate 2-sulfotransferase. Genes Dev 1998;12:1894–1906.
30 Forsberg E, Pejler G, Ringvall M, Lunderius C, Tomasini-Johansson B, Kusche-Gullberg M, Eriksson I, Ledin J, Hellman L, Kjellén L: Abnormal mast cells in mice deficient in a heparin-synthesizing enzyme. Nature 1999, in press.
31 Brickman YG, Ford MD, Gallagher JT, Nurcombe V, Bartlett PF, Turnbull JE: Structural modification of fibroblast growth factor-binding heparan sulfate at a determinative stage of neural development. J Biol Chem 1998;273:4350–4359.
32 Feyzi E, Saldeen T, Larsson E, Lindahl U, Salmivirta M: Age-dependent modulation of heparan sulfate structure and function. J Biol Chem 1998;273:13395–13398.
33 Kreuger J, Prydz K, Pettersson RF, Lindahl U, Salmivirta M: Characterization of fibroblast growth factor 1 binding heparan sulfate domain. Glycobiology 1999;9:723–729.
34 Kinnunen T, Raulo E, Nolo R, Maccarana M, Lindahl U, Rauvala H: Neurite outgrowth in brain neurons induced by heparin-binding growth-associated molecule (HB-GAM) depends on the specific interaction of HB-GAM with heparan sulfate at the cell surface. J Biol Chem 1996;271:2243–2248.
35 Lauri SE, Kaukinen S, Kinnunen T, Ylinen A, Imai S, Kailu K, Taira T, Rauvala H: Regulatory role and molecular interactions of a cell-surface heparan sulfate proteoglycan (N-syndecan) in hippocampal long-term potentiation. J Neurosci 1999;19:1226–1235.
36 Jayson GC, Lyon M, Paraskeva C, Turnbull JE, Deakin JA, Gallagher JT: Heparan sulfate undergoes specific structural changes during the progression from human colon adenoma to carcinoma in vitro. J Biol Chem 1998;273:51–57.
37 Safaiyan F, Lindahl U, Salmivirta M: Selective reduction of 6-O-sulfation in heparan sulfate from transformed mammary epithelial cells. Eur J Biochem 1998;252:576–582.
38 Kjellén L, Bielefeld D, Hook M: Reduced sulfation of liver heparan sulfate in experimentally diabetic rats. Diabetes 1983;32:337–342.
39 Lindahl B, Lindahl U: Amyloid-specific heparan sulfate from human liver and spleen. J Biol Chem 1997;272:26091–26094.
40 Snow AD, Mar H, Nochlin D, Kimata K, Kato M, Suzuki S, Hassell J, Wight TN: The presence of heparan sulfate proteoglycans in the neuritic plaques and congophilic angiopathy in Alzheimer's disease. Am J Pathol 1988;133:456–463.
41 Snow AD, Sekiguchi RT, Nochlin D, Kimata K, Kato M, Suzuki S, Hassell J, Wight TN: Heparan sulfate proteoglycan in diffuse plaques of hippocampus but not of cerebellum in Alzheimer's disease brain. Am J Pathol 1994;144:337–347.
42 Goedert M, Jakes R, Spillantini MG, Hasegawa M, Smith MJ, Crowther RA: Assembly of microtubule-associated protein tau into Alzheimer-like filaments induced by sulfated glycosaminoglycans. Nature 1996;383:550–553.
43 Giulian D, Haverkamp LJ, Yu J, Karshin W, Tom D, Li J, Kanzanskaia A, Kirkpatrick J, Roher AE: The HHQK domain of beta-amyloid provides a structural basis for the immunopathology of Alzheimer's disease. J Biol Chem 1998;273:29719–29726.
44 Koenig A, Norgard-Sumnicht K, Linhardt R, Varki A: Differential interactions of heparin and heparan sulfate glycosaminoglycans with the selectins. J Clin Invest 1998;101:877–889.

Main Paper

Hæmostasis

Haemostasis 1999;29(suppl 1):48–60

The Use of Heparin for Treating Human Malignancies

Deborah L. Ornstein[a] Leo R. Zacharski[b]

[a]Hematology Oncology Flight, Wilford Hall USAF Medical Center, Lackland Air Force Base, San Antonio, Tex., and [b]Veterans Administration Medical Center, White River Junction, Vt., USA

Key Words
Human · Cancer · Heparin · Metastasis

Abstract
There is a substantial amount of data implicating coagulation mechanisms in the pathogenesis of malignancy. Studies in some experimental animal models have shown that the anticoagulant heparin limits tumour growth and metastasis and prolongs survival. Experience with the effects of heparin on human malignancy is limited primarily to settings in which it was given either to prevent or to treat thrombosis in patients who also had cancer. However, these studies have shown noteworthy apparent improvement in cancer outcome with heparin, especially with low-molecular-weight heparin. There are several possible mechanisms by which heparin could potentially alter the natural history of cancer progression because of its ability to modify the cellular and molecular environment of tumour cells. This experience provides the rationale for definitive clinical trials of heparin in patients with cancer and also for further experimentation to define the mechanisms of antineoplastic activity by this familiar class of drugs.

Copyright © 1999 S. Karger AG, Basel

Introduction

Heparin has been studied intensively for decades by scientists interested in its anticoagulant properties. It has several additional activities, however, which seem to have little to do with anticoagulation. In 1930, it was reported that heparin inhibited tumour growth in animals [1], and this led to a period of prolific investigation of its anticancer prop-

KARGER

Fax + 41 61 306 12 34
E-Mail karger@karger.ch
www.karger.com

© 1999 S. Karger AG, Basel
0301–0147/99/0297–0048$17.50/0

Accessible online at:
www.karger.com/journals/hae

Dr . D.L. Ornstein
Hematology Oncology Flight
Wilford Hall USAF Medical Center
59th Medical Wing, Lackland Air Force Base
San Antonio, TX 78227 (USA)

erties. Interest in this field has increased recently with the publication of two meta-analyses of clinical trials comparing the use of unfractionated heparin (UFH) and low-molecular-weight heparin (LMWH) for treatment of venous thromboembolism (VTE) [2, 3]. These analyses demonstrated improved survival for the subset of patients with cancer who received LMWH compared with those who received UFH. The improved outcome was not attributable to prevention of VTE in any study, thus leading to the hypothesis that LMWH may have anticancer activity that is independent of its action as an anticoagulant. This review summarizes animal and human studies on heparin in malignancy and discusses potential mechanisms that account for its antitumour effect.

Investigations in Animals

Goerner was the first to describe the effects of heparin on the progression of experimental malignancy [1]. He found that implanting Flexner-Jobling carcinoma fragments into rats resulted uniformly in the growth of tumours and, eventually, in death of the animals. By contrast, tumour fragments incubated briefly with heparin prior to implantation failed to grow, and all animals who received heparin-treated tumour fragments were alive at 3 months. A period of intensive investigation of anticoagulants and tumour dissemination, spanning more than four decades, began in the 1950s with Terranova and Chiossone, who worked with a rat model of the Walker 256 tumour [4]. Tumour cells were injected intravenously, and metastatic colonies in the lungs were counted at specified time intervals. These workers found that administration of heparin prior to tumour cell inoculation reduced the number of lung colonies and prolonged survival significantly. Studies of the V2 carcinoma in a rabbit ear-chamber model showed that heparin treatment of animals inoculated with tumour cells reduced adhesion of intravascular tumour cells to the vascular endothelium, the motility of tumour cells in tissues and the frequency of metastases [5]. Others demonstrated that V2 carcinoma homogenates possessed thromboplastic properties that rapidly induced intravascular thrombosis and death when injected into rabbits. Death could be prevented by pretreating the animals with heparin [6]. Furthermore, it was shown that heparin also reduced the number of pulmonary metastases and altered the organ distribution of metastatic sites [6, 7].

This pioneering work prepared the way for considerable related experimentation. Although some authors found that heparin delayed the growth of primary tumours [8], most observed that it inhibited metastasis formation [9–13]. Others found that heparin inhibited uptake of radiolabelled fibrinogen into primary tumours [14] and blocked tumour-induced disseminated intravascular coagulation (DIC) in rats [15]. Heparin also prolonged the circulation time of injected tumour cells [16], blocked migration of injected tumour cells from blood vessels to lymphatic channels [17], and inhibited entrapment of tumour cells in pelvic venous plexes following tail injection in rats [18].

Subsequent studies recognized cooperative effects of heparin with other molecules. For example, heparin was shown to potentiate the antitumour effects of alkylating agents, polyinosinic-polycytidylic acid, interferon, tumour necrosis factor and an alpha-2-glycoprotein [19–22]. The metastasis-inhibiting activity of heparin was greatly potentiated by stimulating the reticuloendothelial system with the immunostimulant polidin [23]. In a rat model of human colorectal cancer, there was a trend toward slower tumour growth and longer survival for animals treated with heparin plus 5-fluorouracil (5-FU) compared with those treated with 5-FU alone [24].

Investigations in Humans

The observation that heparin inhibited tumour growth and metastasis in experimental systems was part of a larger body of evidence implicating the blood clotting mechanism in the pathophysiology of cancer. Explanations for the antitumour effects of heparin were usually not apparent from these early studies, however, or they were obscured by differences in animal species, tumour models or other design factors. Despite exhaustive data analysis, a coherent picture of this field that would aid rational clinical trial design failed to emerge, accounting for the fact that early appeals for controlled clinical trials of heparin in cancer patients went unheeded.

Although controlled clinical trials of heparin used specifically to treat cancer have been few in number, heparin has been administered to cancer patients, alone or in combination with other agents, in a variety of other experimental settings. Some of the more stimulating investigations of heparin in cancer patients are summarized in the following discussion.

Several case reports have documented the successful use of heparin to treat cancer [25–28]. The last [28] documents a case of pancreatic cancer in which a partial response to cytotoxic chemotherapy was converted to complete tumour regression by adding heparin to the chemotherapeutic regimen. Although only a single case report, this represents a remarkable result for pancreatic cancer, which is typically refractory to systemic therapy.

Thrombosis occurs frequently in cancer patients, and these patients are often included incidentally in clinical trials of anticoagulants. This has afforded the opportunity to observe the antitumour effect of heparin, albeit indirectly, by looking retrospectively at clinical outcomes in the subgroups of patients with cancer. In one study, medical patients admitted to hospital through the emergency department for reasons other than VTE were randomized to receive or not receive heparin thromboprophylaxis [29]. Overall hospital mortality was reduced by 31% in the heparin-treated group ($p < 0.05$). In the subset of patients with malignancy, overall mortality was reduced by 42% in the heparin-treated group.

Retrospective analyses of studies of colon cancer patients treated with heparin have yielded interesting results. A randomized trial of adjuvant razoxane versus placebo in 603 patients with completely resected colon cancer demonstrated no survival benefit for treatment with razoxane [30]. The investigators observed, however, that some patients received heparin thromboprophylaxis at the same time of surgery while others did not. Retrospective analysis revealed that heparin administration conferred a statistically significant survival advantage to the 329 heparin-treated patients compared with the 274 untreated controls ($p = 0.04$), and this survival advantage was not explained by any other differences between the two groups. The benefit persisted throughout the period of follow-up and was particularly striking for patients with more advanced disease, i.e. stage III tumours. These findings were consistent with those of a previously reported retrospective study of perioperative heparin in colon cancer surgery [31]. In a retrospective study of surgery for all types of cancers, the mortality in 163 patients treated perioperatively with heparin was significantly lower than in 168 untreated patients over the 3-year follow-up period (7.6 versus 12.5%; $p = 0.0005$) [32]. Deaths from metastatic disease occurred in 21.4% of the untreated patients compared with 9.2% of the heparin-treated patients.

LMWH appears to have advantages over UFH for treating VTE in cancer patients. A recent meta-analysis of 13 clinical trials examined the safety and efficacy of LMWH and UFH for treating VTE in unselected patients [3]. The study concluded that LMWH is likely to be more effective for preventing recurrent VTE and less likely to cause serious bleeding than UFH in all patients. In addition, treatment with LMWH appeared to reduce the mortality rate for cancer patients. The relative risk of death at 3 months for LMWH-treated patients was 0.33 (95% CI, 0.1–0.8), a 67% reduction compared with UFH-treated patients (p = 0.01). A reduction in mortality was not evident during the first 15 days of treatment and most patients died after discontinuing heparin treatment, suggesting that the beneficial effect of heparin was not exclusively derived from prevention of recurrent VTE. Whether longer treatment with LMWH would have additional benefit with regard to overall survival in cancer patients is still an open question.

Well-designed prospective trials of heparin for treating cancer are limited. One such small study was reported in 1975 [33]. Twenty-eight patients with inoperable lung cancer who had failed to respond to radiation or chemotherapy were enrolled. The first 14 patients were treated with a combination chemotherapy regimen, which comprised five drugs delivered over a 9-day period, followed by a 2-week rest period. The second group of 14 patients was therapeutically anticoagulated with intravenous heparin for 48 h prior to administering the same chemotherapeutic regimen. Heparin was continued throughout the 9-day treatment period, after which warfarin was substituted for the 2-week rest period. Patients in both groups underwent repeated cycles of treatment until there was definite evidence of tumour progression. No evidence of tumour regression was apparent in any patients in the group receiving chemotherapy only, and all 14 patients died of progressive disease. In the group of patients who received adjunctive heparin, there was a 50% objective response rate, and the response duration ranged from 4 to 18 months. The results of this small study suggest that either heparin has antitumour activity of its own or that it acts synergistically with the chemotherapeutic drugs with which it was combined. Nearly two decades later, a larger study in patients with small-cell lung cancer produced similar results [34]. Patients were randomized to receive (n = 138) or not receive (n = 139) adjusted-dose subcutaneous heparin injections along with combination chemotherapy. Heparin-treated patients demonstrated significantly higher tumour response rates (37 versus 23%; p = 0.004) and median survival (317 versus 261 days; p = 0.01).

Von Tempelhoff and colleagues have reported the results of a prospective double-blind trial comparing UFH and LMWH for thromboprophylaxis in 60 patients undergoing surgery for ovarian cancer [35]. Patients were randomized to receive UFH (n = 32) or LMWH (n = 28) daily until the seventh post-operative day. There were no significant differences in patient characteristics between the two groups, and both groups subsequently received six cycles of adjuvant chemotherapy. The endpoints of the study were the incidence of post-operative VTE and overall survival. There was no difference in VTE incidence between the two groups, but there was a trend toward improved overall survival in the LMWH-treated group, although this did not reach statistical significance. This result is nevertheless encouraging, especially given the small size of the study, and lends support to the observation from meta-analysis that survival in cancer patients may be improved by short-term treatment with LMWH. This study also raises the question of whether patients might have benefited from a more prolonged course of LMWH. This issue should be addressed in future clinical trials.

While the studies of heparin for treating human cancer are provocative, the data remain inconclusive. Prospective large-scale clinical trials that are controlled for tumour type, disease stage and concomitant therapy will be required to test the hypothesis that heparin is an effective anticancer agent in human malignancy.

Potential Mechanisms of the Anticancer Activity of Heparin

Heparin is a highly sulphated member of the glycosaminoglycan (GAG) family, whose other members include heparan sulphate, chondroitin sulphate, dermatan sulphate and keratan sulphate [reviewed in 36–38]. It is found in the mast cells of all mammalian species and is widely distributed throughout a variety of organs. Heparin is synthesized by mast cells in a coordinated, stepwise fashion. A heparin proteoglycan core is generated by the addition of oligosaccharide linkers to serine residues within the polypeptide serglycan, which itself consists of alternating units of serine and glycine. Long polysaccharide chains (approximate molecular weight 100,000 daltons) containing alternating units of N-acetylglucosamine (NAG) and glucuronic acid (GLU) are synthesized by extension of the oligosaccharide linkers. The NAG and GLU residues are enzymatically modified to a variable extent throughout the polysaccharide chains. Up to 80% of the NAG residues are ester-sulphated at the C2 and C6 positions, and the majority of the GLU residues are epimerized to iduronic acid and partially ester-sulphated at the C2 position. The net result of these modifications is an extensively sulphated heparin proteoglycan, containing polysaccharide chains of variable molecular weight (30,000–100,000 daltons). The final step in heparin biosynthesis is degradation of the heparin proteoglycan by lysosomal enzymes to generate highly negatively charged heparin GAG chains with molecular weights ranging from 5,000 to 30,000 daltons.

A discussion of mechanisms of heparin action in cancer must consider effects observed in vitro and in vivo and take into account differences between UFH and LMWH that may explain disparate outcomes in cancer patients treated with these two forms of heparin. Heparins may interact directly with cancer cells or may influence tumours indirectly by associating with proteins and other molecules that subsequently modulate their activity. The factors involved in tumour growth and metastasis and the hypothesized mechanisms by which heparin may act to inhibit each process are reviewed in references 39–41 and summarized in table 1.

Why LMWH May be Better than UFH for Cancer

LMWH [reviewed in 38] is synthesized by limited chemical or enzymatic cleavage of UFH at the unsulphated glucosamine residues. The average molecular mass of LMWH is 4,000–6,000 daltons, compared with 10,000–12,000 daltons for UFH. Both forms of heparin bind to antithrombin (AT) and induce a conformational change that markedly increases its serine-protease-inhibitory activity. The smaller molecules of LMWH, however, have relatively selective inhibitory activity against factor Xa compared with thrombin, the clinical significance of which is currently unknown.

Table 1. Possible mechanisms of heparin effect on tumour growth and metastasis

Mechanisms of tumour growth and metastasis	Potential effects of heparin
Carcinogenesis and tumour growth	
Thrombin is a mitogen for tumour cells, induces the release of VEGF from endothelial cells and platelets, and increases tumour cell adhesiveness [42, 43]	Heparin is an antithrombin [44]
Histamine promotes tumour growth in experimental models [39]	Heparin binds to and inactivates histamine [45]
Chemokines (e.g. IL-8, melanoma growth stimulating factor) stimulate growth and metastasis [45]	Heparin inhibits chemokine activity [46]
Viruses (e.g. EBV, HIV, CMV) are implicated in the pathogenesis of some human tumours	Heparin has antiviral properties [47, 48]
ROS initiate carcinogenesis and promote metastasis [49]	Heparin inhibits ROS production and protects cells from damage by ROS [50, 51]
Oncogenes and transcription factors mediate tumour growth and development [52]	Heparin blocks the expression of certain oncogenes [53, 54]
Casein kinase II is elevated in tumour cell lines and in some human tumours. It may inhibit the activity of the tumour suppressor P53 and/or act as an oncogene [55–57]	Heparin is a potent inhibitor of casein kinase II [58]
Telomerases and topoisomerases are required for cell growth and replication [59, 60]	Heparin may inhibit these enzymes by binding to the positively charged amino acids in the active sites [39]
GAGs in the ECM form a storage depot for cell growth promoting and inhibitory factors and govern their orientation to tumour cell surface receptors [61, 62]	Heparin may alter the collection, activation or transport of tumour growth factors by interacting with GAGs in the ECM [41]
Scatter factor is a tumour cell mitogen [reviewed in 39]	Heparin binds to the cationic clusters in scatter factor and inhibits its activity [63]
Tumour-cell-associated proteoglycans bind to growth factors [64]	Soluble heparin may compete with proteoglycans for growth factor binding [64]
Transcription factors in the AP-1 family are involved in malignant transformation	Heparin inhibits AP-1 binding to DNA [66]
Fibrin is a scaffold for tumour growth, protects tumours from NK cells and participates in angiogenesis [43, 67]	Heparin inhibits fibrin formation [44]
Angiogenesis	
Angiogenesis supports tumour growth [68, 69]	Heparin inhibits angiogenesis [70–72]
TF stimulates angiogenesis [73]	Heparin inhibits TF expression and enhances tissue factor pathway inhibitor [74, 75]
VEGF, IL-8 and hepatocyte growth factor/scatter factor stimulate angiogenesis [76–78]	Heparin is anionic and may bind to the clusters of basic amino acids in these proteins and inhibit their activity [reviewed in 39]
VEGF binding to the KDR/flk-1 receptor complex requires a positively charged amino acid surface [79]	Heparin is highly negatively charged and may interfere with binding and, therefore, angiogenesis

➤

Table 1 (continued)

Mechanisms of tumour growth and metastasis	Potential effects of heparin
Tumour adhesion, invasion, metastasis	
Tumour adhesion to vascular endothelial cell surfaces is a critical step in metastasis [81]	Heparin binds to and may inactivate molecules involved in adhesion (e.g. selectins and heparan sulphate proteoglycans) and alter the adhesive properties of tumour and endothelial cells [82, 83]
Complement promotes metastasis in experimental models [84]	Heparin inhibits the classical and alternative pathways of complement activation [85]
MMPs facilitate metastasis [86]	Heparin could bind to the highly positively charged active sites of MMPs and inhibit their activity [reviewed in 39]
Thrombin and plasminogen activators can activate MMP [86]	Heparin inhibits thrombin and plasminogen activators, and could thus inhibit MMP activity indirectly [44]
Thrombospondin facilitates migration, attachment and spreading of tumour cells [87]	Heparin can inhibit thrombospondin binding to receptors [88]
Serine proteases (e.g. thrombin, urokinase, plasmin, cathepsin G) stimulate tumour growth metastasis [89]	Heparin inhibits the activity of these enzymes, possibly by binding to the positively charged active sites [90, 91]
Protease nexin is a serine protease inhibitor (serpin) that blocks tumour cell invasion [92]	Heparin binds to protease nexin and accelerates its linkage to substrates, as well as activates other serpins [93, 94]
Heparanase degrades basement membranes, and its expression correlates with the metastatic potential of some tumour cells [95]	Heparin blocks tumour cell heparanases and decreases tumour metastases in experimental models [96]
Ornithine decarboxylase is a cationic enzyme that catalyses polyamine biosynthesis. Its overexpression increases the invasiveness of epithelial cell tumours [97]	Heparin is anionic and may inhibit ornithine decarboxylase activity [reviewed in 39]
Antineoplastic factors	
TGF-β may have antineoplastic effects [reviewed in 39]	Heparin potentiates TGF-β activity in some experimental systems [98–100]
Malignant cells have lost the capacity for apoptosis	Heparin induces apoptosis in some experimental tumours [101, 102]
Malignant cells have lost the ability to differentiate	Heparin induces differentiation of some experimental tumours [103]
Immunosuppression enhances the growth of some human cancers	Heparin stimulates lymphocyte reactivity and cytoxic antitumour responses in some experimental systems [104, 105]
Expression of MDR proteins by leukaemia cells renders them resistant to killing by chemotherapeutic drugs	Heparin reverses the MDR phenotype in various leukaemia cell lines [106]

AP-1 = Activating protein-1; ECM = extracellular matrix; MDR = multidrug resistance; MMP = metalloproteinase; NK = natural killer; ROS = reactive oxygen species; TF = tissue factor; TGF-β = transforming growth factor β; VEGF = vascular endothelial growth factor.

Table 2. Differences between LMWH and UFH with implications for treating cancer patients

Compared with UFH, LMWH has	Possible advantages of LMWH over UFH for cancer treatment
More inhibitory effect on angiogenesis and on basic fibroblast growth factor (b-FGF)-induced proliferation of colon cancer cells [107–109]	More potent anticancer activity
Less platelet-activating activity [110]	Less production of thrombin and other tumour growth factors
Less ability to mediate vascular permeability [111]	May limit tumour egress from the intravascular space
Less binding to plasma proteins [112]	Predictable pharmacokinetics and safe, convenient daily dosing without monitoring
Less binding to von Willebrand factor [112]	Less interference with interactions between platelets and blood vessel walls, and fewer bleeding complications
Less interaction with platelet factor 4 [113, 114]	Lower incidence of heparin-induced thrombocytopenia and thrombosis
Less associated osteoclast activation [115]	Potential for less osteopenia/osteoporosis with long-term use
Stimulatory effect on megakaryopoiesis and platelet production [116]	May attenuate chemotherapy-induced thrombocytopenia

LMWH exhibits less binding to plasma proteins and cell surfaces, which results in better bioavailability and a longer half-life than UFH, and accounts for its dose-dependent clearance. In addition, multiple animal and clinical studies have shown that LMWH is at least as effective as UFH as an anticoagulant but with less associated bleeding. The improved toxicity profile of LMWH may be due to reduced binding to von Willebrand factor, platelets and endothelial cells, and thus less interference with interactions between platelets and blood vessel walls. Because of its superior pharmacokinetic properties, LMWH can be administered subcutaneously in a fixed dose without laboratory monitoring, making it safer and more convenient to administer to outpatients than UFH.

LMWH and UFH differ in a number of other important respects, which have been reviewed extensively [38]. Although there is a paucity of comparative data, there is nevertheless some evidence that LMWH has more anticancer activity than UFH. The mechanisms responsible for this observation are not known but may be related to differential effects of LMWH and UFH on angiogenesis, tumour growth factors and/or metastatic processes. Moreover, there are some characteristics of LMWH unrelated to its antitumour activity that make it appealing for use in cancer patients, whose diseases are often terminal and for whom quality of life is greatly enhanced by treatments that maximize time spent out of the hospital and clinic. Table 2 summarizes the differences between LMWH and UFH that may have implications for treating cancer patients. This is an active area of investigation, which is evolving rapidly, and there are likely to be continual additions to this list.

Conclusions

The evidence that heparin has anticancer activity in human malignancy, while currently inconclusive, is nevertheless provocative. The abundance of preclinical data in this area supports the idea that there may be an important role for heparin in the treatment of cancer and provides the rationale for further testing in humans. The widespread availability of a safer and more conveniently administered formulation of heparin, i.e. LMWH, makes such studies more feasible than ever before.

The hypothesis that heparin improves survival in cancer patients is relatively easily tested in prospective, randomized clinical trials. These studies must be designed specifically to assess the effect of heparin on cancer, independently of the effect of other treatments including chemotherapy, radiation and surgery. The preferred trial design is that which has been previously employed by others, in which patients with a single tumour type are randomized to receive accepted, standard antineoplastic therapy for that tumour type with or without added heparin [33, 34]. The advantage of conducting separate clinical trials for each different tumour type is that one is able to control for differences in the biology of different tumours that may affect the efficacy of heparin. Most likely, human cancers will demonstrate a heterogeneous response to heparin based on the specific biology of individual tumour types, and clinical trials may ultimately show that heparin is effective only in certain tumour types. LMWH is the clear choice for these studies because of its superior pharmacokinetics, efficacy and convenience, and lower toxicity, compared with UFH. The optimum dose, schedule and length of administration of LMWH remain to be determined, however.

Clinical trials will also provide a setting for studies of mechanisms. As we have suggested in this review, heparin may alter the natural history of malignancy by numerous pathways. Current technology should allow many of these to be studied directly, and comparative studies of LMWH and UFH in cancer may provide important clues to the underlying mechanisms of both tumour growth and the inhibition of growth. Existing data on heparin effects in human malignancy provide a starting point for future studies, but there is much work still to be done.

References

1 Goerner A: The influence of anticlotting agents on transplantation and growth of tumor tissue. J Lab Clin Med 1930;16:369–372.
2 Lensing A, Prins M, Davidson B, Hirsh J: Treatment of deep venous thrombosis with low molecular weight heparins. A meta-analyis. Arch Intern Med 1995;155:601–607.
3 Siragusa S, Cosmi B, Piovella F, Hirsh J, Ginsburg J: Low-molecular-weight heparins and unfractionated heparin in the treatment of patients with acute venous thromboembolism: Results of a meta-analysis. Am J Med 1996;100:269–277.
4 Terranova T, Chiossone F: The coagulation factor in the attachment of neoplastic cells introduced into the blood stream. Boll Soc Ital Biol Sper 1952;28:1224–1225.
5 Wood S Jr, Holyoke E, Yardley J: An experimental study of the influence of adrenal steroids, growth hormone and anticoagulants on pulmonary metastasis formation in mice. Proc Am Assoc Cancer Res 1956;2:157–158.
6 Lawrence E, Bowman D, Moore D, Bernstein G: A thromboplastic property of neoplasms. Surg Forum 1952;3:394–398.
7 Lawrence E, Moore D, Bernstein G: The ability of the pulmonary vascular system to influence the spread of tumor emboli. J Thorac Surg 1953; 26:233–240.
8 Kudrjaskov B, Kalishevskaya T, Kolomina S: Blood anticoagulating system and malignant tumours. Nature 1969;222:548–550.

9 Fisher B: Experimental studies of factors which influence hepatic metastases. VIII. Effects of anticoagulants. Surgery 1961;50:240–247.
10 Agostino D, Cliffton E: Anticoagulants and the development of pulmonary metastases. Arch Surg 1962; 84:449–453.
11 Ivarsson L, Rudenstam C-M: Heparin, dextran 1000 and metastasis formation after IV tumour cell injection in dextran non-sensitive rats. Br J Cancer 1975;32:502–508.
12 Owen CJ: Anticoagulant treatment of rats with Walker 256 carcinosarcomas. J Cancer Res Clin Oncol 1982;104:191–193.
13 Drago J, Weed P, Fralisch A: The evaluation of heparin in control of metastasis of Nb rat androgen-insensitive prostate carcinoma. Anticancer Res 1984;4:171–172.
14 Shaeffer J: Interference in localization of 131-iodine fibrinogen in rat tumors by anticoagulants. Am J Physiol 1964;206:573–579.
15 Heyes H, Kohle W: Heparin-dependent inhibition of microangiopathic haemolytic anaemia in an experimental rat tumour. Thromb Haemost 1979;42:240.
16 Koike A: Mechanism of blood-borne metastases. I. Some factors affecting lodgment and growth of tumor cells in the lungs. Cancer 1964; 17:450–460.
17 Hilgard P, Beyerle L, Hohage R, Hiemeyer V, Kubler M: The effect of heparin on the intitial phase of metastasis formation. Eur J Cancer 1972;8:347–352.
18 van den Brenk H, Burch W, Kelly H, Orton C: Venous diversion trapping and growth of blood-borne cancer cells en route to the lungs. Br J Cancer 1975;3:46–61.
19 Saba T, Cho E: Alteration of tumor growth by a purified alpha-2-glycoprotein. J Reticuloendothelial Soc 1977;22:583–596.
20 Csaba G, Korosi J, Horvath C, Mold K, Acs T: Effect of heparin-bound alkylating agents and enzyme inhibitors on neoplastic growth. Neoplasma 1964;11:137–143.
21 Lee A, Rogers L, Longcroft J, Jeffery R: Reduction of metastasis in a murine mammary tumor model by heparin and polyinosinic-polycytidylic acid. Clin Exp Metast 1990;8:165–171.
22 Sylvester D, Liu Y, Meadows G: Augmentation of antimetastatic activity of interferon and tumor necrosis factor by heparin. Immunopharmacol Immunotoxicol 1990;12: 161–180.
23 Kiricuta I, Todorutiu C, Muresian T, Risca R: Prophylaxis of metastasis formation by unspecific immunologic stimulation associated with heparin therapy. Cancer 1973;31: 1392–1396.
24 Nagawa H, Paris P, Chauffert B, Martin F: Treatment of experimental liver metastasis in the rat by continuous intraportal infusion of 5-fluorouracil and heparin: A pilot study. Anticancer Drugs 1990;1: 149–156.
25 Albert-Weil J, Nehorais J: A propos de deux cas de néoplasies non justiciable des therapeutiques classiques, traitées per des injections intraveineuses d'héparine et des injections intramusculaires d'un extrait de sangsue. Rev Pathol Gén Comparée 1954;54:1014–1020.
26 Astedt B, Glifberg I, Mattsson W, Trope C: Arrest of growth of ovarian tumor by tranexamic acid. J Am Med Assoc 1977;238:154–155.
27 Astedt B, Mattsson W, Trope C: Treatment of advanced breast cancer with chemotherapeutics and inhibition of coagulation and fibrinolysis. Acta Med Scand 1977;201: 491–493.
28 Sadoff L, Latino F: Complete clinical remission in a patient using mitomycin C-based chemotherapy: The role of adjunctive heparin. Am J Clin Oncol 1999;22:187–190.
29 Halkin H, Goldberg J, Modan M, Modan B: Reduction of mortality in general medicine inpatients by low-dose heparin prophylaxis. Ann Intern Med 1982;96:561–565.
30 Kingston R, Fielding J, Palmer M: Peri-operative heparin: A possible adjuvant to surgery in colo-rectal cancer? Int J Colorect Dis 1993;8: 111–115.
31 Tongren S, Rieger A: The influence of heparin and curable resection on the survival of colon cancer. Acta Chir Scand 1983;149:427–429.
32 Kakkar A, Hedges A, Williamson R, Kakkar V: Perioperative heparin therapy inhibits late death from metastatic cancer. Int J Oncol 1995; 6:885–888.
33 Elias E, Shulka S, Mink I: Heparin and chemotherapy in the management of inoperable lung cancer. Cancer 1975;36:129–136.
34 Lebeau B, Chastang C, Brechot J-M, Capron F, Dautzenberg B, Delaisements C, Mornet M, Brun J, Hurdebourcq J-P, Lemarie E: Subcutaneous heparin treatment increases survival in small cell lung cancer. Cancer 1994;74:38–45.
35 von Tempelhoff G-F, Dietrich M, Neimann F, Schneider D, Hommel G, Heilmann L: Blood coagulation and thrombosis in patients with ovarian malignancy. Thromb Haemost 1997;77:456–461.
36 Kjellen L, Lindahl U: Proteoglycans: Structures and interactions. Ann Rev Biochem 1991;60:443–475.
37 Iozzo R: Proteoglycans: Structure, function and role in neoplasia. Lab Invest 1985;53:373–396.
38 Weitz J: Low molecular weight heparins. N Engl J Med 1997;337:688–698.
39 Engelberg H: Actions of heparin that may affect the malignant process. Cancer 1999;85:257–272.
40 Hejna M, Raderer M, Zielinski C: Inhibition of metastases by anticoagulants. J Natl Cancer Inst 1999; 91:22–36.
41 Zacharski L, Ornstein D: Heparin and cancer. Thromb Haemost 1998; 80:10–23.
42 Mohle R, Green D, Moore M, Nachman R, Rafii S: Constitutive production and thrombin-induced release of vascular endothelial growth factor by human megakaryocytes and platelets. Proc Natl Acad Sci USA 1997;94:663–668.
43 Markus G: The role of haemostasis and fibrinolysis in the metastatic spread of cancer. Thromb Haemost 1984;10:61–72.
44 Hirsh J: Heparin. N Engl J Med 1991;324:1565–1574.
45 Engelberg H: Evidence that endogenous heparin activity deficiency may be an important factor in atherogenesis. Semin Thromb Hemost 1997;23:159–166.
46 Miller M, Krangel M: Biology and biochemistry of the chemokines: A family of chemotactic and inflammatory cytokines. Crit Rev Immunol 1992;12:17–46.

47 Howell A, Taylor T, Miller J, Groveman D, Eccles E, Zacharski L: Inhibition of HIV-1 infectivity by low molecular weight heparin. Results of in vitro studies and a pilot clinical trial in patients with advanced AIDS. Int J Clin Lab Res 1996;26:124–131.
48 Hosoya M, Balzirini J, Shigeta S, DeClerq E: Differential inhibitory effects of sulfated polysaccharides and polymers on the replication of various myxoviruses and retroviruses depending on the composition of the target amino acid sequences of the viral envelope glycoproteins. Antimicrob Agents Chemother 1991;35:2515–2520.
49 Lesko S, Lorentzen R, Tso P: Role of superoxide in deoxyribonucleic acid strand scission. Biochemistry 1980;19:3023–3028.
50 Hiebert L, Lui J: Heparin protects cultured arterial endothelial cells from damage by toxic oxygen metabolites. Atherosclerosis 1990;83:47–51.
51 Hladovec J: Protective effect of oxygen-derived free radical scavengers on the endothelium in vivo. Physiol Bohemoslov 1986;35:97–103.
52 Land H, Parada L, Weinberg R: Cellular oncogenes and multistep carcinogenesis. Science 1983;62:771–778.
53 Wang A, Templeton D: Inhibition of mitogenesis and c-fos induction in mesangial cells by heparin and heparan sulfates. Kidney Int 1996;49:437–448.
54 Bennett M, Evan G, Newby A: Deregulated expression of the c-myc oncogene abolishes inhibition of proliferation of rat vascular smooth muscle cells by serum reduction, interferon-gamma, heparin and cyclic nucleotide analogues and induces apoptosis. Circ Res 1994;74:525–536.
55 Muganda P, Fischer A, Bernal R: Identification of a casein kinase activity found elevated in human cytomegalovirus transformed cells. Biochem Biophys Res Commun 1995;207:740–746.
56 Seldin D, Leder P: Casein kinase IIa transgene-induced murine lymphoma: Relation to theileriosis in cattle. Science 1995;267:894–897.
57 Filhol O, Boudier J, Delphin C, Loue-Mackenbach P, Chambaz E, Cochet C: Casein kinase II and the tumor suppressor protein p53 associate in a molecular complex that is negatively regulated upon p53 phosphorylation. J Biol Chem 1992;267:20577–20583.
58 Hathaway G, Lubben T, Traugh J: Inhibition of casein kinase II by heparin. J Biol Chem 1980;255:8038–8041.
59 Wang J: DNA topoisomerases. Ann Rev Biochem 1996;65:635–692.
60 Feng J, Funk W, Wang S: The RNA component of human telomerase. Science 1995;269:1236–1241.
61 Buddecke E: Non-anticoagulant functions of heparin and heparan sulfate. Hamostaseologie 1996;16:15–24.
62 Zimmerman J, Bar-Shavit R, Peretz T, Ben-Sasson S: Control of cell proliferation by heparan sulfate and heparin-binding growth factors. Thromb Haemost 1995;74:534–540.
63 Mizuno K, Inoue H, Hagiya M, Shimizu S, Noar T, Shimohigashi Y, Nakamura T: Hairpin loop and second kringle domain are essential sites for heparin binding and biological activity of hepatocyte growth factor. J Biol Chem 1994;269:1131–1136.
64 Ruoslahti E, Yamaguchi Y: Proteoglycans as modulators of growth factor activities. Cell 1991;64:867–869.
65 Smeal T, Binstroy B, Mercola D, Birrer M, Karin M: Oncogenic and transcriptional cooperation with Ha-Ras requires phosphorylation of c-Jun on serines 63 and 73. Nature 1990;354:494–496.
66 Au Y, Dobrowolska G, Morris D, Clowes A: Heparin decreases activator protein-1 binding to DNA in part by posttranslational modification of Jun B. Circ Res 1994;75:15–22.
67 Gungi Y, Gorelik E: Role of fibrin coagulation in protection of murine tumor cells from destruction by cytotoxic cells. Cancer Res 1988;48:5216–5221.
68 Folkman J: Clinical applications of research on angiogenesis. N Engl J Med 1995;333:1757–1763.
69 Weidner N, Semple J, Welch W, Folkman J: Tumour angiogenesis and metastasis – correlation in invasive breast carcinoma. N Engl J Med 1991;324:1–8.
70 Derbyshire E, Comin G, Yang Y, Overholser J, Watkins L, Thorpe P: Anti-tumor and anti-angiogenic effects in mice of heparin conjugated to angiostatic steroids. Int J Cancer 1995;63:694–701.
71 Folkman J, Langer R, Linhardt R, Haudenschild C, Taylor S: Angiogenesis inhibition and tumor regression caused by heparin or a heparin fragment in the presence of cortisone. Science 1983;221:719–725.
72 Jacobson A, Hahnenberger R: Antiangiogenic effect of heparin and other sulfated glycosaminoglycans in the chick embryo chorioallantoic membrane. Pharmacol Toxicol 1991;69:122–126.
73 Zhang Y, Deng Y, Luther T, Miller M, Ziegler R, Waldher R, Stern D, Nawroth P: Tissue factor controls the balance of angiogenic and antiangiogenic properties of tumor cells in mice. J Clin Invest 1994;94:1320–1327.
74 Pepe G, Guisti B, Attanasio M, Gori A, Comeglio P, Martini F, Gensini G, Abbate R, Neri Serneri G: Tissue factor and plasminogen activator inhibitor type 2 expression in human stimulated monocytes is inhibited by heparin. Semin Thromb Hemost 1997;23:135–141.
75 Jeske W, Fareed J, Eschenfelder V, Iqbal O, Hoppensteadt D, Ashan A: Biochemical and pharmacologic characteristics of reviparin, a low-molecular-mass heparin. Semin Thromb Hemost 1997;23:119–128.
76 Arenberg D, Kunkel S, Polverini P, Glass M, Burdick M, Streiter R: Inhibition of interleukin-8 reduces tumorigenesis of human non-small cell lung cancer in SCID mice. J Clin Invest 1996;97:2792–2802.
77 Camussi G, Montrucchio G, Lupia E, Soldi R, Conoglio P, Bussolino F: Angiogenesis induced in vivo by hepatocyte growth factor is moderated by platelet activating factor synthesis from macrophages. J Immunol 1997;158:1302–1309.

78 Claffey K, Brown L, del Aquila L, Tognazzi K, Yen K, Manseau E, Dvorak H: Expression of vascular permeability factor/vascular endothelial cell growth factor by melanoma cells increases tumor growth, angiogenesis and experimental metastasis. Cancer Res 1996;56:172–181.
79 Keyt B, Nguyen H, Berleau L, Duarte C, Park J, Chen H, Ferrara N: Identification of VEGF determinants for binding KDR and FLT-1 receptors: Generation of receptor-selective VEGF variants. J Biol Chem 1996;271:5638–5646.
80 Jackson R, Busch S, Cardin A: Glycosaminoglycans: Molecular properties, protein interactions, and role in physiological processes. Physiol Rev 1991;71:481–539.
81 Springer T: Traffic signals for lymphocyte recirculation and leukocyte emigration: The multistep paradigm. Cell 1994;76:301–314.
82 Nelson R, Cecconi O, Roberts W, Aruffo A, Lindhardt R, Bavilacqua M: Heparin oligosaccharides bind L- and P-selectin and inhibit acute inflammation. Blood 1993;82: 3253–3258.
83 Norgard-Sunnicht K, Varki N, Varki A: Calcium dependent heparin-like ligands for L-selectin in nonlymphoid endothelial cells. Science 1993;261:480–483.
84 Orr F, Adamson I, Young L: Pulmonary inflammation generates chemotactic activity for tumor cells and promotes lung metastasis. Am Rev Resp Dis 1985;131:607–611.
85 Engelberg H: Actions of heparin in the atherosclerotic process. Pharmacol Rev 1996;48:327–352.
86 Stetler-Stevenson W, Hewitt R, Corcoran M: Matrix-metalloproteases and tumor invasion: From correlation and causality to the clinic. Semin Cancer Biol 1996;7:147–154.
87 Tuszynski G, Smith M, Rothman V, Capuzzi D, Joseph R, Katz J, Besa E, Treat J, Switalska H: Thrombospondin levels in patients with malignancy. Thromb Haemost 1992; 67:607–611.
88 Schon P, Vischer P, Volker W, Schmidt A, Faver V: Cell associated proteoheparan sulfate mediates binding and uptake of thrombospondin in cultured porcine vascular endothelial cells. Eur J Cell Biol 1992;59:329–339.
89 Schmitt M, Harbeck N, Thomssen C, Wilhelm O, Magdolen V, Reuning U, Ulm K, Hofler H, Janicke F, Graeff H: Clinical aspects of the plasminogen activation system in tumor invasion and metastasis: Prognostic relevance and target for therapy. Thromb Haemost 1997;78: 285–296.
90 Jeske W, Fareed J: Antithrombin III- and heparin cofactor II-mediated anticoagulant and antiprotease actions of heparin and its synthetic analogues. Semin Thromb Hemost 1993;19(suppl 1):241–247.
91 Pratt C, Tobin R, Church F: Interaction of heparin cofactor II with neutrophil elastase and cathepsin G. J Biol Chem 1990;265:6092–6097.
92 Farrell D, Cunningham D: Human fibroblasts accelerate the inhibition of thrombin by protease nexin. Proc Natl Acad Sci 1981;83:6858–6862.
93 Hermans J, Monard D, Jones R, Stone S: Inhibition of acrosin by serpins. A suicide substrate mechanism. Biochemistry 1995;34:3678–3685.
94 Low D, Baker J, Koon W, Cunningham D: Released protease nexin regulates cellular binding, internalization and degradation of serine proteases. Proc Natl Acad Sci USA 1981;78:2340–2344.
95 Bitan M, Mohsen M, Levi E: Structural requirements for inhibition of melanoma lung colonization by heparanase inhibitory species of heparin. Isr J Med Sci 1995;31:106–118.
96 Parish C, Coombe D, Jacobsen K, Bennett F, Underwood P: Evidence that sulfated polysaccharides inhibit tumor metastases by blocking tumor cell-derived heparanases. Int J Cancer 1987;40:511–518.
97 Smith M, Goral M, Wright J, Matrisian L, Morris R, Klein-Szanto A, Gilmour S: Ornithine decarboxylase overexpression leads to increased epithelial tumor invasiveness. Cancer Res 1997;57:2104–2108.
98 McCaffrey T, Falcone D, Vicente D, Du B, Consigli S, Borth W: Protection of transforming growth factor-beta 1 activity by heparin and fucoidan. J Cell Physiol 1994;159: 356–361.
99 Knaus P, Lindemann D, Decoteau J, Perlman R, Hillerta MY: A dominant inhibitory mutant of the type II transforming growth factor beta receptor in the malignant progression of a cutaneous T cell lymphoma. Mol Cell Biol 1996;16: 3480–3489.
100 Garrigua-Antar L, Muñoz-Antonia T, Antonia S, Gesmonde J, Villuci V, Reise M: Missense mutations of the transforming growth factor beta type II receptor in human head and neck squamous carcinoma cells. Cancer Res 1995;55: 3982–3987.
101 Granerus M, Engstrom W: Growth factors and apoptosis. Cell Prolif 1996;29:309–314.
102 Manaster J, Chezar J, Shurtz-Swirski R, Shapiro G, Tendler Y, Kirstal B, Shasha S, Sela S: Heparin induces apoptosis in human peripheral blood neutrophils. Br J Haematol 1996;94:48–52.
103 Luikart S, Maniglia C, Furcht L, McCarthy J, Oegema T Jr: A heparan sulfate-containing fraction of bone marrow stroma induces maturation of HL-60 cells in vitro. Cancer Res 1990;50:3781–3785.
104 Dziarski R: Enhancement of mixed leukocyte reaction and cytotoxic antitumor responses by heparin. J Immunol 1989;143:356–365.
105 Eskinazi D, Perna J, Ershow A, Sharrow S: Effects of heparin on in vivo immune parameters. J Biol Response Mod 1988;7:173–184.
106 Maia R, Wagner K, Cabral R, Rumjanek V: Heparin reverses rhodamine 123 extrusion by multidrug resistant cells. Cancer Lett 1996;106:101–108.
107 Norrby K, Ostergaard P: Basic fibroblast growth factor-mediated de-novo angiogenesis is more effectively suppressed by low molecular weight heparin than by high molecular weight heparin. Int J Microcirc Clin Exp 1996;16:8–15.

108 Jayson G, Gallagher J: Heparin oligosaccharides: Inhibitors of the biological activity of bFGF on Caco2 cells. Br J Cancer 1997;75: 9–16.
109 Norrby K: Heparin and angiogenesis: A low-molecular-weight fraction inhibits and a high-molecular-weight fraction stimulates angiogenesis. Haemostasis 1993; 23(suppl 1):141–149.
110 Salzman E, Rosenberg R, Smith M, Lindon J, Favreau L: Effect of heparin and heparin fragments on platelet aggregation. J Clin Invest 1980;65:64–73.
111 Blajchman M, Young E, Ofosu F: Effects of unfractionated heparin, dermatan sulfate and low molecular weight heparin on vessel wall permeability in rabbits. Ann NY Acad Sci 1989;556:245–254.
112 Cosmi B, Fredenburgh J, Rischke J, Hirsh J, Young E, Weitz J: Effect of nonspecific binding to plasma proteins on the antithrombin activities of unfractionated heparin, low molecular weight heparin and dermatan sulfate. Circulation 1997;95:118–124.
113 Kelton J, Smith J, Warkentin T, Hayward C, Denomme G, Horsewood P: Immunoglobin G from patients with heparin-induced thrombocytopenia binds to a complex of heparin and platelet factor 4. Blood 1994;83:3232–3239.
114 Lane D, Denton J, Flynn A, Thunberg L, Lindahl U: Anticoagulant activities of heparin oligosaccharides and their neutralization by platelet factor 4. Biochem J 1984; 218:725.
115 Muir J, Hirsh J, Weitz J, Andrew M, Young E, Shaughnessy S: A histomorphometric comparison of the effects of heparin and low-molecular-weight heparin on cancellous bone in rats. Blood 1997;89: 3236–3242.
116 Shen Z, Basara N, Xi X, Caen J, Maffrand J, Pascal M, Petiton M, Lormeau J, Han Z: Fraxiparin, a low-molecular-weight heparin, stimulates megakaryocytopoiesis in vitro and in vivo in mice. Br J Haematol 1994;88:608–612.

Main Paper

Hæmostasis

Haemostasis 1999;29(suppl 1):61–67

Heparins in Diabetic Microangiopathy: Rationale and Preliminary Clinical Results

Fokko J. van der Woude

Vth Medical University Clinic, Klinikum Mannheim, Germany

Key Words
Heparins · Heparan sulphate · Microangiopathy · Diabetes nephropathy · Glycosaminoglycans

Abstract
It has been postulated, based upon epidemiological data, that genetic differences in the enzymes involved in the sulphation of glycosaminoglycan (GAG) side-chains of heparan sulphate (HS) proteoglycans are of crucial importance in the pathogenesis of diabetic nephropathy. An alteration in GAG metabolism is also believed to be responsible for the well-known co-occurrence of diabetic nephropathy and extrarenal micro- and macroangiopathy. In this article, recent in-vitro and in-vivo studies on the role of HS-GAG in the pathogenesis of diabetic nephropathy are discussed. Preliminary data suggest that HS-GAG treatment may be of benefit in patients with insulin-dependent diabetes mellitus, nephropathy and retinopathy. Results in patients with non-insulin-dependent diabetes mellitus are less convincing, although not completely negative.

Copyright © 1999 S. Karger AG, Basel

The notion that heparan sulphate proteoglycans (HSPGs) and/or other heparin-like substances could be of significant importance in diabetic microangiopathy comes from studies of diabetic nephropathy.

Epidemiology

Diabetic nephropathy has become one of the main causes of end-stage renal disease in the Western world; the latest incidence figures among patients starting on dialysis vary from 16% in the Netherlands [1] to 42% in the USA [2]. Consequently, not only is the disease very expensive, it also has a large impact in terms

KARGER
Fax + 41 61 306 12 34
E-Mail karger@karger.ch
www.karger.com

© 1999 S. Karger AG, Basel
0301–0147/99/0297–0061$17.50/0

Accessible online at:
www.karger.com/journals/hae

Dr. F.J. van der Woude
Vth Medical University Clinic
Klinikum Mannheim, Ruperto Carola University, Heidelberg
Theodor-Kutzer-Ufer 1–3
D–68135 Mannheim (Germany)

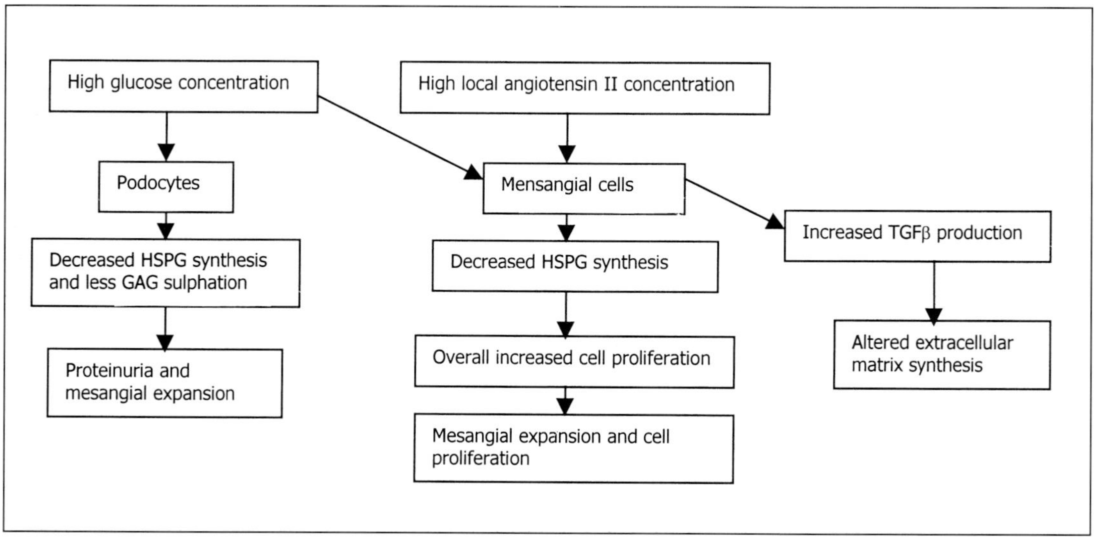

Fig. 1. Synopsis of the possible pivotal role of HSPG in the pathogenesis of the glomerular alteration in diabetic nephropathy. There are insufficient data on glomerular endothelial cells in this respect, and these cells are, therefore, not depicted in this diagram.

of associated morbidity and mortality for the individual patient [3]. The pathogenesis of diabetic nephropathy is complex; hyperglycaemia (see figure 1) [4], blood pressure regulation [5, 6] and genetic factors [7–10] all play an important role. Albuminuria and proteinuria are the most important risk factors predicting cardiovascular mortality in patients with diabetes mellitus [11, 12]. One of the many theories developed to explain this association is the Steno hypothesis. This hypothesis, which was first developed by Deckert et al. in 1988, proposes that a genetic defect in the regulation of the production of heparan sulphate (HS) by endothelial cells, vascular smooth muscle cells and mesangial cells determines the susceptibility of diabetic patients to develop proteinuria and angiopathy, with its associated cardiovascular risk [13]. Playing a central role in this hypothesis is the sulphation pattern of the glycosaminoglycan (GAG) side-chains of HSPGs. Deckert and colleagues postulated that diabetic patients, susceptible to nephropathy and macroangiopathy, have a genetic trait leading to a lower activity of the enzymes responsible for GAG sulphation under high glucose conditions. The resulting undersulphated GAG chains could then play a crucial role in the pathogenesis of proteinuria and its morphological substrate diabetic nephropathy, as well as in the pathogenesis of diabetic micro- and macroangiopathy. Although genes have been cloned for N-deacetylase/N-sulphotransferase, for 3-sulphotransferase and for 6-O-sulphotransferase enzymes [for review, see 14], it is presently unclear whether different allotypes of such enzymes, with different susceptibilities to high glucose concentrations, really exist. Although the Steno hypothesis clearly has not been formally proven, it has certainly been fruitful for in-vitro experiments and therapeutic trials in experimental animals and patients.

Pathophysiology

Biochemical studies using ^{35}S sulphate incorporation have shown a decreased basement membrane HSPG production in diabetic glomeruli in experimental animal models, and direct chemical analysis of human tissues obtained postmortem has revealed a decreased GAG content of kidneys and aortas of patients with diabetic nephropathy [for review, see 15].

A decreased presence of glomerular basement membrane (GBM) HSPG expression was shown in tissue with mesangial expansion in diabetic nephropathy with a technique where histochemical staining with cuprolinic blue was combined with electron microscopy morphometry [16]. In the last decade, new monoclonal antibodies against GAG chains and core proteins of various HSPGs have become available [17]. A very interesting antibody, JM-403, reacting with HS-GAG chains, mainly stains the GBM in normal kidneys and largely fails to stain tubular basement membranes. The epitope recognized by this monoclonal antibody contains one or more N-unsubstituted glucosamine and D-glucuronic acid units and is located in a region of the HS chain composed of mixed N-sulphated and N-acetylated disaccharide units [18]. With this antibody, it was shown that a decreased GBM staining intensity correlated with proteinuria, expressed as a function of creatinine clearance, in patients with diabetic nephropathy [19]. It was also shown that staining of skin basement membrane with JM-403 was significantly reduced in patients with diabetic nephropathy as compared with patients with long-standing diabetes without nephropathy [20]. It should be noted that the exact meaning of a decreased staining of this antibody under pathologic conditions with regard to total GAG content or sulphation is not yet known. The first major basal membrane HSPG to be identified was perlecan [21]; results of immunohistological staining in diabetic nephropathy with antibodies against HSPG core proteins did not reveal any significant changes [17, 19]. To date, three HSPG core proteins have been identified in the GBM: perlecan, agrin [22] and collagen XVIII (which is a collagen and proteoglycan) [23]. Interestingly, domain-specific monoclonal antibodies revealed a differential expression of agrin in glomerular and tubular basement membranes, suggesting alternative splicing and/or post-translational processing of the molecule within the kidney [24]. Agrin is only present in the kidney and the nervous system, and studies on agrin metabolism in diabetes are currently in progress.

The effects of the diabetic milieu on glomerular HSPG synthesis have been studied in vitro using glomerular cell cultures [for review, see 25]. In studies using human glomerular visceral epithelial and mesangial cells cultured under normal (5 mM) and high (25 mM) glucose conditions, staining with JM-403 – i.e. the same monoclonal antibody as used on the tissue sections of diabetic kidneys – revealed a decreased extracellular matrix staining after culturing in high glucose [25]. An altered proteoglycan production under high glucose conditions was also observed using metabolic labelling, with predominantly a decrease in HSPG as compared with dermatan or chondroitin sulphate proteoglycan. N-sulphation analysis of HSPG produced under high glucose conditions revealed less di- and tetrasaccharides as compared with larger oligosaccharides, indicating an altered sulphation pattern.

Renal function deterioration and proteinuria in diabetic patients are correlated with mesangial expansion as the main morphological parameter [26]. Since angiotensin-converting-enzyme inhibitors are known to slow the progression of diabetic nephropathy [5] and since we were interested in the role of HSPG in diabetic nephropathy, we studied the effect of angiotensin II (Ang II) on mesangial HSPG production. In addition, as Ang II is known to stimulate extracellular matrix production through transforming-growth-factor-β (TGF-β) production in rat mesangial cells [27], we also studied the role of TGF-β in this regard [28]. Metabolic labelling studies revealed that Ang II induced a decrease of HSPG synthesis, with decreases in N-sulphation of the GAG side-chains. ELISA measurements using JM-403 confirmed that Ang II decreased HS production. Ang II increased TGF-β production in a dose-dependent fashion. Specific mRNA for perlecan HSPG decreased, while mRNA for TGF-β increased, after incubation with Ang II. Blockade of the subtype-1 Ang II receptor (ATR1) reversed the effects of Ang II on both HSPG and TGF-β production. Co-incubation of the mesangial cells with neutralizing antibodies against TGF-β significantly reduced the production of HS as compared with controls and Ang II. These results indicate that the decrease in HS synthesis induced by Ang II is not mediated by an increase in TGF-β; on the contrary, the increase in TGF-β partially counteracts the inhibition of HS production by Ang II.

Since defects in HS-GAG synthesis are so prominently present in in-vitro models of diabetic nephropathy (induced by either high glucose concentrations or Ang II), and since decreased renal and extrarenal JM-403 staining seems to be a rather specific marker for nephropathy in patients with diabetes, treatment of diabetic nephropathy with HS-GAG-like substances can be seen as an experiment to test the Steno hypothesis.

Therapeutic Studies

Numerous reports have shown that heparin and, more generally, GAGs prevent and cure experimental diabetic nephropathy [29–33]. Several hypotheses have been formulated to explain the renoprotective effect of heparin and GAGs in experimental diabetes: down-regulation of proteases, modulation of extracellular mesangial matrix synthesis, and restoration of GBM anionic charges [for review, see 34, 35]. Recently, these favourable results in animal models have been partially confirmed in human disease. Indeed, recent reports have described favourable results of GAG treatment on proteinuria in diabetic nephropathy. Treatment with a low-molecular-weight heparin reduced urinary albumin excretion in patients with insulin-dependent diabetes mellitus (IDDM) and either micro- or macroalbuminuria [36, 37]. Furthermore, danaparoid, a mixture of sulphated GAGs consisting mainly of HS, was shown to lower proteinuria in a small, double-blind, cross-over study in IDDM patients with albumin excretion rates higher than 300 mg/24 h [38]. It was at least 6 weeks before the anti-proteinuric effect manifested itself, without effects on blood pressure and creatinine clearance. Sulodexide, a formulation composed of two GAGs (80% fast-moving heparin and 20% dermatan sulphate), has been reported to reduce albuminuria in patients with IDDM or non-insulin-dependent diabetes mellitus (NIDDM) [39–42], with the effect lasting for several weeks after withdrawal [40, 43]. Although sulodexide treatment seems always to be effective in reducing microalbuminuria in IDDM, the hypoalbuminuric effect is seen in only 33–50% of NIDDM patients. In a recently performed, randomized, placebo-controlled parallel study with danaparoid sodium (750 anti-Xa units once daily) in 22 NIDDM patients, no changes in urinary albumin or protein excretion were found [44]. It is known that microalbuminuria in NIDDM patients is not always caused by diabetic nephropathy, since two-thirds of patients have been reported to have different, non-diabetic histological changes [45]. The studies published to date have been too short to clarify whether GAG treatment is capable of curing diabetic nephropathy rather than simply influencing one of its surrogate endpoints, albuminuria.

One major point of concern about the use of GAGs and heparin in the treatment of diabetic patients has been the risk of bleeding, particularly in subjects with retinal neoangiogenesis, due to the fragility of new vessels. Although the dosages used were relatively small, sufficient only to inhibit factor X, we recently demonstrated therapy with the GAG danaparoid to be safe in IDDM patients [46]. Even more interesting, the data showed a reduction of retinal hard exudates. This was a surprising observation, since it is known that a spontaneous reduction of such abnormalities is not likely to occur within a few months. How can these findings be explained?

Overexpressed vascular endothelial growth factor (VEGF) plays a pivotal role in diabetic retinopathy, both the proliferative form and maculopathy [47]. Interestingly, in physiological conditions, some VEGF isoforms are sequestered, and modulated by extracellular matrix sulphated GAGs. Alterations of the sulphation of GAGs in diabetes could thus lead to an altered disposal of VEGF, and exogenous GAGs might revert this phenomenon [48]. Thus, the effect of danaparoid on hard exudates might well be related to the modulation of sequestered VEGF in the retina. In NIDDM patients, the favourable effect of danaparoid treatment on retinopathy could not be confirmed [44].

Conclusions

The Steno hypothesis postulates a crucial role for heparin-like structures in the pathogenesis of diabetic nephropathy. Although the epidemiology of diabetic nephropathy and retinopathy are very different, clinical data now suggest that treatment with heparin or heparin-like substances may be of benefit in both conditions, at least in IDDM patients. Although these data are rather incompatible with the Steno hypothesis, they do suggest that the GAG chains of heparin molecules have some specific structures that are useful for renal and retinal protection. These specific structures need not necessarily have a relationship with the anticoagulant activity of heparin. Further studies are needed, not only to confirm and extend the data (e.g. dose-finding studies are missing), but also to define better the exact clinical and functional conditions in diabetic nephropathy that are treatable with heparins. Last but not least, we still have to show that, in humans, not only surrogate endpoints like proteinuria and retinal exudates, but also renal function, vision and morphological abnormalities, can be improved.

References

1 Renine Foundation: De ontwikkeling van het nierfunctie-vervangingsprogramma in Nederland. Statistisch verslag. Rotterdam, Erasmus University Rotterdam, 1998.
2 The 'United States Renal Data System' is available on: URL: http://www.med.umich.edu/usrds. Chapter II: Incidence and prevalence of ESRD, 1999.
3 Pastan S, Bailey J: Dialysis therapy. N Engl J Med 1998;338:1428–1437.
4 DCCT Research Group: The effect of intensive treatment of diabetes on the development and progression of long-term complications in insulin-dependent diabetes mellitus. N Engl J Med 1993;329:977–986.
5 Lewis EJ, Hunsicker LG, Bain RP, Rohde RD: The effect of angiotensin-converting-enzyme inhibition on diabetic nephropathy. N Engl J Med 1993;329:1456–1462.
6 Mogensen CE: How to protect the kidney in diabetic patients. Diabetes 1997;46(suppl 2):S104–S111.
7 Seaquist ER, Goetz FC, Rich S, Barbosa J: Familial clustering of diabetic kidney disease. Evidence for genetic susceptibility to diabetic nephropathy. N Engl J Med 1989;320:1161–1165.
8 Pettitt DJ, Nelson RG, Saad MF, Bennett PH, Knowler WC: Diabetes and obesity in the offspring of Pima Indian women with diabetes during pregnancy. Diabetes Care 1993;16:310–314.
9 Borch-Johnsen K, Norgaard K, Hommel E, Mathiesen ER, Jensen JS, Deckert T, Parving HH: Is diabetic nephropathy an inherited complication? Kidney Int 1991;41:719–722.
10 Parving HH, Tarnow L, Rossing P: Genetics of diabetic nephropathy. J Am Soc Nephrol 1996;7:2509–2517.
11 Parving HH, Osterby R, Anderson PW, Hsueh W: Diabetic nephropathy; in Brenner BM (ed): The Kidney, ed 5. Philadelphia, Saunders, 1996, pp 1864–1892.
12 Rossing P, Hougaard P, Borch-Johnsen K, Parving HH: Predictors of mortality in insulin dependent diabetes: 10 year observational follow-up study. BMJ 1996;313:779–784.
13 Deckert T, Feldt-Rasmussen B, Borch-Johnsen K, Kofoed-Enevoldsen A: Albuminuria reflects widespread vascular damage. The Steno hypothesis. Diabetologia 1989;32:219–226.
14 Rosenberg RD, Shworak NW, Liu J, Schwartz JJ, Zhang L: Heparan sulfate proteoglycans of the cardiovascular system. Specific structures emerge but how is synthesis regulated? J Clin Invest 1997;100:S67–S75.
15 Van der Woude FJ, van Det NF: Heparan sulphate proteoglycans and diabetic nephropathy. Exp Nephrol 1997;5:180–188.
16 Vernier RL, Steffes MW, Sissons-Ross S, Mauer M: Heparan sulfate proteoglycan in the glomerular basement membrane in type I diabetes mellitus. Kidney Int 1992;41:1070–1080.
17 Van den Born J, van den Heuvel LPWJ, Bakker MAH, Veerkamp JH, Assman KJM, Weening JJ, Berden JHM: Distribution of GBM heparan sulfate proteoglycan core protein and side chains in human glomerular diseases. Kidney Int 1993;43:454–463.
18 Van den Born J, Gunnarson K, Bakker MAH, Kjellen L, Kusche-Gullberg M, Maccarana M, Berden JHM, Lindahl U: Presence of N-unsubstituted glucosamine units in native heparan sulfate revealed by a monoclonal antibody. J Biol Chem 1995;270:31303–31309.
19 Tamsma JT, van den Born J, Bruijn JA, Assmann KJM, Weening JJ, Berden JHM, Wieslander J, Schrama E, Hermans J, Veerkamp JH, Lemkes HHPJ, van der Woude FJ: Expression of glomerular extracellular matrix components in human diabetic nephropathy: Decrease of heparan sulphate in the glomerular basement membrane. Diabetologia 1994;37:313–320.
20 Van der Pijl JW, Daha MR, van den Born J, Verhagen NA, Lemkes HH, Bucala R, Berden JH, Zwinderman AH, Bruijn JA, van Es LA, van der Woude FJ: Extracellular matrix in human diabetic nephropathy: Reduced expression of heparan sulphate in skin basement membrane. Diabetologia 1998;41:791–798.
21 Iozzo RV, Cohen IR, Grässel S, Murdoch AD: The biology of perlecan: The multifaceted heparan sulphate proteoglycan of basement membranes and pericellular matrices. Biochem J 1994;302:625–639.
22 Groffen AJ, Ruegg MA, Dijkman H, van de Velden TJ, Buskens CA, van den Born J, Assmann KJ, Monnens LA, Veerkamp JH, van den Heuvel LP: Agrin is a major heparan sulfate proteoglycan in the human glomerular basement membrane. J Histochem Cytochem 1998;46:19–27.
23 Halfter W, Dong S, Schurer B, Cole GJ: Collagen XVIII is a basement membrane heparan sulfate proteoglycan. J Biol Chem 1998;273:25404–25412.
24 Raats CJ, Bakker MA, Hoch W, Tamboer WP, Groffen AJ, van den Heuvel LP, Berden JH, van den Born J: Differential expression of agrin in renal basement membranes as revealed by domain-specific antibodies. J Biol Chem 1998;273:17832–17838.
25 Van Det NF, van den Born J, Tamsma JT, Verhagen NAM, Berden JHM, Bruijn JA, Daha MR, van der Woude FJ: Effects of high glucose on the production of heparan sulfate proteoglycan by human mesangial and glomerular visceral epithelial cells in vitro. Kidney Int 1996;49:1079–1089.
26 Mauer SM, Steffes MW, Ellis EN, Sutherland DE, Brown DM, Goetz FC: Structural-functional relationships in diabetic nephropathy. J Clin Invest 1984;74:1143–1155.

27 Kagami S, Border WA, Miller DA, Noble NA: Angiotensin II stimulates extracellular matrix protein synthesis through induction of transforming growth factor-β expression in rat glomerular mesangial cells. J Clin Invest 1994;93:2431–2437.
28 van Det NF, Tamsma JT, van den Born J, Verhagen NAM, van den Heuvel LPWJ, Lowik CWGM, Berden JHM, Bruijn JA, Daha MR, van der Woude FJ: Differential effects of angiotensin II and transforming growth factor β on the production of heparan sulfate proteoglycan by mesangial cells in vitro. J Am Soc Nephrol 1996;7:1015–1023.
29 Gambaro G, Venturini AP, Noonan DM, Fries W, Re G, Garbisa S, Milanesi C, Pesarini A, Borsatti A, Marchi E, Baggio B: Treatment with a glycosaminoglycan formulation ameliorates experimental diabetic nephropathy. Kidney Int 1994;46:797–806.
30 Gambaro G, Cavazzana AO, Luzi P, Piccoli A, Borsatti A, Crepaldi G, Marchi E, Venturini AP, Baggio B: Glycosaminoglycans prevent morphological renal alterations and albuminuria in diabetic rats. Kidney Int 1992;42:285–291.
31 Ceol M, Nerlich A, Baggio B, Anglani F, Sauer U, Schleicher E, Gambaro G: Increased glomerular α1(IV) collagen expression and deposition in long-term diabetic rats is prevented by chronic glycosaminoglycan treatment. Lab Invest 1996;74:484–495.
32 Oshima Y, Isogai S, Mogama K, Ohuchi H, Ohe K: Protective effect of heparin on renal glomerular anionic sites of streptozotocin-injected rats. Diab Res Clin Pract 1995;25:83–89.
33 Oturai PS, Rasch R, Hasseleger E, Johansen PB, Yokoyama H, Thomsen MK, Myrup B, Kofoed-Enevoldsen A, Deckert T: Effects of heparin and aminoguanidine on glomerular basement membrane thickening in diabetic rats. Acta Pathol Microbiol Scand 1996;104:259–264.
34 Gambaro G, Baggio B: Glycosaminoglycans: A new paradigm in the prevention of proteinuria and progression of glomerular disease. Nephrol Dial Transplant 1996;11:762–764.
35 Gambaro G, Barbanti M, Marchi E, Baggio B: Therapy with glycosaminoglycans in nephrology; in Harenberg J, Casu B (eds): Nonanticoagulant Actions of Glycosaminoglycans. New York, Plenum Press, 1996, pp 281–286.
36 Myrup B, Hansen PM, Jensen T, Kofoed-Enevoldsen A, Feldt-Rasmussen B, Gram J, Kluft C, Jespersen J, Deckert T: Effect of low-dose heparin on urinary albumin excretion in insulin-dependent diabetes mellitus. Lancet 1995;345:421–422.
37 Tamsma JT, van der Woude FJ, Lemkes HHPJ: Effect of sulfated glycosaminoglycans on albuminuria in patients with overt diabetic (type-1) nephropathy. Nephrol Dial Transplant 1996;11:182–185.
38 Van der Pijl JW, van der Woude FJ, Geelhoed-Duijvestijn PHLM, Fröhlich M, van der Meer FJM, Lemkes HHPJ, van Es LA: Danaparoid sodium lowers proteinuria in diabetic nephropathy. J Am Soc Nephrol 1997;8:456–462.
39 Solini A, Carraro A, Barzon I, Crepaldi G: Therapy with glycosaminoglycans lowers albumin excretion rate in non-insulin-dependent diabetic patients with microalbuminuria. Diab Nutr Metab 1994;7:304–307.
40 Skrha J, Perusicova J, Pontuch P, Oksa A: Glycosaminoglycan sulodexide decreases albuminuria in diabetic patients. Diab Res Clin Pract 1997;38:25–31.
41 Poplawska A, Szelachowska M, Topolska J, Wysocka-Solowie B, Kinalska I: Effect of glycosaminoglycans on urinary albumin excretion in insulin-dependent diabetic patients with micro- or macroalbuminuria. Diab Res Clin Pract 1997;38:109–114.
42 Dedov I, Shestakova M, Vorontzov A, Palazzini E: A randomized, controlled study of sulodexide therapy for the treatment of diabetic nephropathy. Nephrol Dial Transplant 1997;12:2295–2300.
43 Poplawska A, Toplska J, Kinalska I, Grimaldi M: A pilot study of the effect of the glycosaminoglycan sulodexide on microalbuminuria in type I diabetic patients. Curr Med Res Opin 1997;13:539–545.
44 Van der Pijl JW, Lemkes HHPJ, Fröhlich M, van der Woude FJ, van der Meer FJM, van Es LA: Effect of danaparoid sodium on proteinuria, von Willebrand factor, and hard exudates in patients with diabetes mellitus type II. J Am Soc Nephrol 1999;10:1331–1336.
45 Fioretto P, Mauer M, Brocco E: Patterns of renal injury in NIDDM patients with microalbuminuria. Diabetologia 1995;39:1569–1576.
46 Van der Pijl JW, van der Woude FJ, Swart W, van Es LA, Lemkes HHPJ: Effect of danaparoid sodium on hard exudates in diabetic retinopathy. Lancet 1997;350:1743–1745.
47 Paques M, Massin P, Gaudric A: Growth factors and diabetic retinopathy. Diabet Metabol 1997;23:125–130.
48 Klein R, Klein BEK: Diabetic eye disease. Lancet 1997;350:197–204.

Workshop 1 Chairman: J.I. Weitz
New Antithrombotic Drugs: Beyond Aspirin and Heparin

Hæmostasis

Haemostasis 1999;29(suppl 1):68

New Antithrombotic Drugs: Beyond Aspirin and Heparin

Chairman's Summary

Jeffrey I. Weitz

Hamilton Civic Hospitals Research Centre, Hamilton, Ont., Canada

Most acute coronary syndromes are caused by disruption of atherosclerotic plaque with superimposed thrombosis. Coronary artery thrombosis is a thrombin-mediated, platelet-dependent process that is relatively resistant to inhibition by aspirin and heparin. Resistance to aspirin likely reflects the fact that aspirin inhibits only thromboxane-A_2-dependent platelet activation. The thienopyridines (ticlopidine and clopidogrel) also inhibit only a single pathway of platelet activation, by irreversibly blocking the ADP receptor on platelets. Consequently, the thienopyridines provide little additional benefit over aspirin. In contrast, by targeting the final common pathway of platelet aggregation, glycoprotein (GP) IIb/IIIa antagonists block platelet aggregation in response to all agonists. Abciximab, a chimeric Fab fragment directed against GPIIb/IIIa, is of proven efficacy in patients undergoing percutaneous coronary interventions. Likewise, synthetic GPIIb/IIIa antagonists such as tirofiban and eptifibatide are promising agents for the treatment of patients with unstable angina and non-Q-wave myocardial infarction (MI).

Resistance of coronary artery thrombosis to heparin likely reflects the inability of the heparin/antithrombin complex to inactivate thrombin bound to fibrin. By simultaneously binding to thrombin and fibrin, heparin augments and heightens thrombin's interaction with fibrin and renders it resistant to inactivation by antithrombin and heparin cofactor II. In contrast, fibrin-bound thrombin is susceptible to inactivation by direct thrombin inhibitors, such as hirudin and bivalirudin. These agents, which interact with exosite 1 and the active site of thrombin, compete with fibrin for thrombin binding and inactivate both fibrin-bound and fluid-phase thrombin. This may explain why hirudin was better than heparin in patients with unstable angina and non-Q-wave MI, and bivalirudin was superior to heparin in high-risk patients undergoing coronary angioplasty.

KARGER

Fax + 41 61 306 12 34
E-Mail karger@karger.ch
www.karger.com

© 1999 S. Karger AG, Basel
0301–0147/99/0297–0068$17.50/0

Accessible online at:
www.karger.com/journals/hae

Workshop 1

Hæmostasis

Haemostasis 1999;29(suppl 1):69–71

Use of Glycoprotein IIb/IIIa Inhibitors in Patients with Acute Coronary Syndromes Undergoing Coronary Revascularization

Jeffrey J. Popma

Departments of Internal Medicine (Cardiology Division), Brigham and Women's Hospital, Boston, Mass., USA

Key Words
Acute coronary syndromes · Glycoprotein IIb/IIIa inhibitors

Abstract
This paper briefly reviews the results from three recent large-scale clinical trials evaluating the benefit of glycoprotein IIb/IIIa inhibitors in patients with acute coronary syndromes (ACS). The available data suggest that these are promising agents for the management of ACS, particularly in improving the immediate outcome in the acute setting.

Copyright © 1999 S. Karger AG, Basel

Acute coronary syndromes (ACS), i.e. non-Q-wave myocardial infarction (MI) and unstable angina, remain major causes of morbidity and mortality in patients with atherosclerotic coronary artery disease. It has been suggested that glycoprotein (GP) IIb/IIIa inhibitors may be of particular benefit in several subgroups of patients with unstable angina. These subgroups include those with pain when they are at rest, after a recent MI, or despite medical therapy [1]; those with ischaemic ST-segment depressions or T-wave changes in association with pain [2–5]; and those with elevated markers of myocardial necrosis, including creatine kinase monobasic (CK-MB) [6], troponin I [7, 8] and troponin T [8–14].

Three studies have evaluated the effect of 'upstream' use of GPIIb/IIIa inhibition in patients with ACS (table 1). In the CAPTURE (c7E3 Antiplatelet Therapy in Unstable Refractory Angina) study [15], 1,265 patients with refractory unstable angina and planned coronary intervention were randomly assigned to treatment with aspirin plus intravenous heparin or to aspirin plus intravenous heparin plus abciximab bolus (0.25 mg/kg) and infusion (10 μg/h) for 18–24 h prior to the procedure. The 30-day primary endpoint –

KARGER

Fax + 41 61 306 12 34
E-Mail karger@karger.ch
www.karger.com

© 1999 S. Karger AG, Basel
0301–0147/99/0297–0069$17.50/0

Accessible online at:
www.karger.com/journals/hae

Dr. Jeffrey J. Popma
Departments of Internal Medicine (Cardiology Division)
75 Francis Street
Boston, MA 02115 (USA)

Table 1. Summary of clinical trials evaluating GP IIb/IIIa inhibitors in patients with ACS

Clinical trial	Year	Patients	Treatment
CAPTURE [15]	1997	1,265	Aspirin + heparin or aspirin + intravenous heparin + abciximab
PURSUIT [16]	1998	10,948	Aspirin + placebo or aspirin+ heparin + eptifibatide
PRISM-PLUS [17]	1998	1,570	Heparin or heparin + tirofiban

CAPTURE = c7E3 Antiplatelet Therapy in Unstable Refractory Angina; PRISM-PLUS = Platelet Receptor Inhibition for Ischemic Syndrome Management in Patients Limited by Unstable Signs and Symptoms; PURSUIT = Platelet Glycoprotein IIb/IIIa in Unstable Angina: Receptor Suppression Using Integrelin Therapy.

comprising death from any cause, MI or the need for urgent intervention due to recurrent ischaemia – occurred in 11.3% of patients who received abciximab and in 15.9% of those given placebo (p = 0.012). This difference was chiefly due to a reduction in MI in abciximab-treated patients before (0.6 vs. 2.1%, respectively; p = 0.029) and after (2.6 vs. 5.5%, respectively; p = 0.009) coronary intervention.

The PURSUIT (Platelet Glycoprotein IIb/IIIa in Unstable Angina: Receptor Suppression Using Integrelin Therapy) trial [16] randomly assigned 10,948 patients with ischaemic chest pain and electrocardiographic changes or elevated serum levels of CK-MB to receive aspirin plus placebo or aspirin plus heparin plus eptifibatide for 72 h. Compared with the placebo group, those treated with eptifibatide had a 1.5% absolute reduction in the incidence of the primary 30-day composite endpoint of death and non-fatal MI (14.2 vs. 15.7% in the placebo group; p = 0.04). Coronary intervention was performed in 1,228 patients within 72 h of randomization. In those patients undergoing coronary intervention, there was a 31% reduction in the frequency of 30-day death or non-fatal MI in patients treated with eptifibatide (11.6 vs. 16.7% in placebo-treated patients; p = 0.01).

In the PRISM-PLUS (Platelet Receptor Inhibition for Ischemic Syndrome Management in Patients Limited by Unstable Signs and Symptoms) trial [17], 1,570 patients with unstable angina or non-Q-wave MI were randomly assigned to receive an infusion of heparin alone or heparin plus tirofiban for 48–108 h. Coronary intervention was performed in 30.5% of patients between 48 and 96 h after enrollment. The 30-day composite endpoint of death, MI and recurrent ischaemia was lower in patients treated with heparin plus tirofiban (8.8 vs. 15.3% in patients treated with heparin alone; p = 0.06).

Current evidence suggests that all patients presenting with unstable angina or non-Q-wave MI should be admitted and promptly treated with medications that have proven prognostic benefits, including aspirin, heparin, beta-blockers and, in selected cases, GPIIb/IIIa inhibitors (i.e. abciximab, tirofiban or eptifibatide).

References

1 Braunwald E: Unstable angina. A classification. Circulation 1989;80: 410–414.
2 Haze K, Nonogi H, Miyazaki S, Ito A, Daikoku S: Pathogenesis, treatment and prognosis of impending myocardial infarction and early post-infarction angina – relation between ST-segment shift during myocardial ischemia and the pathogenesis. Jpn Circ J 1992;56:1150–1159.
3 Cannon CP, McCabe CH, Stone PH, Rogers WJ, Schactman M, Thompson BW, Pearce DJ, Diver DJ, Kells C, Feldman T, Williams M, Gibson RS, Kronenberg MW, Ganz LI, Anderson HV, Braunwald E: The electrocardiogram predicts one-year outcome of patients with unstable angina and non-Q wave myocardial infarction: Results of the TIMI III Registry ECG Ancillary Study. Thrombolysis in Myocardial Ischemia. J Am Coll Cardiol 1997; 30:133–140.
4 Betriu A, Heras M, Cohen M, Fuster V: Unstable angina: outcome according to clinical presentation. J Am Coll Cardiol 1992;19:1659–1663.
5 Sclarovsky S, Rechavia E, Strasberg B, Sagie A, Bassevich R, Kusniec J, Mager A, Agmon J: Unstable angina: ST segment depression with positive versus negative T wave deflections – clinical course, ECG evolution, and angiographic correlation. Am Heart J 1988;116:933–941.
6 Markenvard J, Dellborg M, Jagenburg R, Swedberg K: The predictive value of CKMB mass concentration in unstable angina pectoris: Preliminary report. J Intern Med 1992;231: 433–436.
7 Galvani M, Ottani F, Ferrini D, Ladenson JH, Destro A, Baccos D, Rusticali F, Jaffe AS: Prognostic influence of elevated values of cardiac troponin I in patients with unstable angina. Circulation 1997;95:2053–2059.
8 Luscher MS, Thygesen K, Ravkilde J, Heickendorff L: Applicability of cardiac troponin T and I for early risk stratification in unstable coronary artery disease. TRIM Study Group. Thrombin Inhibition in Myocardial Ischemia. Circulation 1997;96:2578–2585.
9 Antman EM, Sacks DB, Rifai N, McCabe CH, Cannon CP, Braunwald E: Time to positivity of a rapid bedside assay for cardiac-specific troponin T predicts prognosis in acute coronary syndromes: A Thrombolysis in Myocardial Infarction (TIMI) IIA substudy. J Am Coll Cardiol 1998;31:326–330.
10 Gokhan Cin V, Gok H, Kaptanoglu B: The prognostic value of serum troponin T in unstable angina. Int J Cardiol 1996;53:237–244.
11 Kerr GD, Dunt DR: Early prediction of risk in patients with suspected unstable angina using serum troponin T. Aust NZ J Med 1997; 27:554–560.
12 Lindahl B, Venge P, Wallentin L: Relation between troponin T and the risk of subsequent cardiac events in unstable coronary artery disease. The FRISC study group. Circulation 1996;93:1651–1657.
13 Solymoss BC, Bourassa MG, Wesolowska E, Dryda I, Theroux P, Mondor L, Perrault D, Gilfix BM: The role of cardiac troponin T and other new biochemical markers in evaluation and risk stratification of patients with acute chest pain syndromes. Clin Cardiol 1997;20:934–942.
14 Stubbs P, Collinson P, Moseley D, Greenwood T, Noble M: Prospective study of the role of cardiac troponin T in patients admitted with unstable angina. Br Med J 1996; 313:262–264.
15 The CAPTURE Investigators: Randomised placebo-controlled trial of abciximab before and during coronary intervention in refractory unstable angina: The CAPTURE study. Lancet 1997;349:1429–1435.
16 The PURSUIT Investigators: Inhibition of platelet glycoprotein IIb/IIIa with eptifibatide in patients with acute coronary syndromes. N Engl J Med 1998;339:436–443.
17 The PRISM-PLUS Investigators: Inhibition of the platelet glycoprotein IIb/IIIa receptor with tirofiban in unstable angina and non-Q-wave myocardial infarction. N Engl J Med 1998;338:1488–1497.

Workshop 1 Chairman: J.I. Weitz
New Antithrombotic Drugs: Beyond Aspirin and Heparin

Hæmostasis

Haemostasis 1999;29(suppl 1):72–75

Low-Molecular-Weight Heparins in Acute Unstable Coronary Artery Disease – An Update

Alexander G.G. Turpie

Department of Medicine, McMaster University, Hamilton, Ont., Canada

Key Words
Unstable angina · Antithrombotic therapy · Low-molecular-weight heparin

Abstract
Low-molecular-weight heparins (LMWHs) have been rigorously evaluated in the management of acute coronary ischaemia. The results of clinical trials suggest that the LMWHs (enoxaparin, dalteparin and nadroparin) are effective and safe in the treatment of unstable angina and non-Q-wave myocardial infarction. Two studies have shown enoxaparin to be more effective than unfractionated heparin in this setting. Furthermore, the pharmacologic and pharmacokinetic characteristics of LMWHs result in them having practical and economic advantages. Data on the benefits of long-term therapy with LMWHs are conflicting.

Copyright © 1999 S. Karger AG, Basel

Antithrombotic therapy with or without revascularization has been extensively studied in patients with acute coronary ischaemic syndromes. The role of aspirin in reducing both fatal and non-fatal myocardial infarction (MI) in the acute phase of unstable angina is well established. Furthermore, the long-term risk of death or MI in patients with acute coronary syndromes is reduced by approximately 50% with regular aspirin use [1]. In acute transmural MI, aspirin alone reduces mortality by 25% [1].

Anticoagulants such as heparin play a key role in inhibiting the generation of thrombin, the enzyme that is central for the formation of fibrin. In patients with unstable angina and non-Q-wave MI, heparin has been shown to decrease the frequency of MI and to reduce overall mortality, particularly when used in combination with aspirin [2–6]. Standard heparin has a number of limitations, however.

KARGER

Fax + 41 61 306 12 34
E-Mail karger@karger.ch
www.karger.com

© 1999 S. Karger AG, Basel
0301–0147/99/0297–0072$17.50/0

Accessible online at:
www.karger.com/journals/hae

Dr. A.G.G. Turpie
HHSC-General Division
237 Barton Street East
Hamilton, Ont., L8L 2X2 (Canada)

Table 1. Summary of LMWH studies/trials

Study	Year	Drug used	Compared with
Gurfinkel et al. [8]	1995	Nadroparin	Aspirin or standard aspirin and heparin
Wallentin et al. (FRISC) [9]	1996	Dalteparin	Aspirin
Klein et al. (FRIC) [10]	1997	Dalteparin	Intravenous unfractionated heparin
Cohen et al. (ESSENCE) [11]	1997	Enoxaparin	Standard heparin
Antman (TIMI 11B) [12]	1997	Enoxaparin	Heparin
Leizorovicz (FRAXIS) [13]	1998	Nadroparin	Heparin
FRISC II [14]	1999	Dalteparin	Placebo Invasive versus non-invasive strategy

ESSENCE = Efficacy and Safety of Subcutaneous Enoxaparin in Non-Q-Wave Coronary Events; FRAXIS = Fraxiparine in Ischaemic Syndromes; FRIC = Fragmin in Unstable Coronary Artery Disease; FRISC = Fragmin During Instability in Coronary Artery Disease; TIMI = Thrombolysis in Myocardial Infarction.

In particular, its anticoagulant effect is unpredictable and it has a poor bioavailability when given subcutaneously. Low-molecular-weight heparins (LMWHs) offer a number of pharmacologic and pharmacokinetic advantages over standard heparin: a predictable anticoagulant response, a high bioavailability and a long plasma half-life, which together result in a therapeutic anticoagulant effect with once- or twice-daily subcutaneous injections at fixed, weight-adjusted doses [7].

A number of LMWHs – enoxaparin, dalteparin and nadroparin – have been evaluated in patients with unstable angina and non-Q-wave MI (table 1). In a small open trial, nadroparin reduced the risk of ischaemic outcomes, as compared with aspirin alone or a combination of aspirin and standard heparin, in the acute phase [8]. Two large trials have evaluated dalteparin in the management of unstable angina and non-Q-wave MI [9, 10]. In the placebo-controlled FRISC trial (Fragmin During Instability in Coronary Artery Disease), dalteparin (120 units/kg subcutaneously twice daily) resulted in a 63% reduction in the risk of death or acute MI, as compared with aspirin alone, in the acute phase, and was associated with a significant reduction in cardiac events at 42 days when it was continued at a dose of 7,500 units subcutaneously once daily [9]. The FRIC trial (Fragmin in Unstable Coronary Artery Disease), which directly compared dalteparin with intravenous unfractionated heparin, demonstrated that dalteparin, administered at the same therapeutic dose, was not significantly different from heparin in the acute phase. Furthermore, this trial, unlike FRISC, showed no benefit of continued treatment with dalteparin at a low dose once daily [10]. In the ESSENCE (Efficacy and Safety of Subcutaneous Enoxaparin in Non-Q-Wave Coronary Events) study [11], involving 3,171 patients, enoxaparin (1 mg/kg subcutaneously twice daily) resulted in a statistically significant 16% reduction in the combined outcome of death, MI and recurrence of angina at 14 and 30 days relative to standard heparin, a benefit that was maintained at 1 year of follow-up.

Recently, three major clinical trials evaluating LMWH in acute coronary ischaemic syndromes have been completed. TIMI (Thrombolysis in Myocardial Infarction) [12] confirmed that enoxaparin was more effective than heparin in the acute phase of treatment of unstable angina and non-Q-wave MI, but did not show any additional benefit of continuing treatment. FRAX.I.S (Fraxiparine in Ischaemic Syndromes) [13] showed no difference in efficacy between nadroparin given for 6 days or 14 days and heparin given for 6 days. FRISC (Fragmin During Instability in Coronary Artery Disease) II [14] evaluated an invasive versus a non-invasive strategy in patients who were initially treated with dalteparin; in addition, it compared dalteparin in therapeutic doses with placebo long term. The study demonstrated superiority of the invasive over the non-invasive strategy and a significant reduction in death and MI at 40 days with dalteparin compared with placebo. However, this latter benefit was attenuated and not statistically significant at 90 days.

The available data indicate that LMWHs are effective and safe in reducing major ischaemic outcomes in patients with unstable angina and non-Q-wave MI. In addition, as LMWHs can be given by fixed-dose subcutaneous injection without monitoring, this results in major cost-savings [15]. Thus, LMWHs represent an important advance in the management of acute non-ST-segment elevation coronary ischaemia and are recommended for this indication in the 1998 American College of Chest Physicians' Guidelines on Antithrombotic Therapy [16].

References

1 ISIS-2 (Second International Study of Infarct Survival) Collaborative Group: Randomised trial of intravenous streptokinase, oral aspirin, both, or neither among 17,187 cases of suspected acute myocardial infarction: ISIS-2. Lancet 1988;ii: 349–360.

2 Theroux P, Omit H, Micas J, Latter J-G, Jolly P, Levy G, Polluter E, Juneau M, Stasis J, Degauss P, Polluter GB, Rinzler D, Waters DD: Aspirin, heparin or both to treat acute unstable angina. N Engl J Med 1988;319:1105–1111.

3 The RISC Group: Risk of myocardial infarction and death during treatment with low dose aspirin and intravenous heparin in men with unstable coronary artery disease. Lancet 1990;336:827–830.

4 Theroux P, Waters D, Qui S, McCans J, deGuise P, Juneau M: Aspirin versus heparin to prevent myocardial infarction during the acute phase of unstable angina. Circulation 1993;88:2045–2048.

5 Theroux P, Waters D, Lam J, Juneau M, McCans J: Reactivation of unstable angina after the discontinuation of heparin. N Engl J Med 1992;327:142–145.

6 Cohen M, Adams PC, Parry G, Xiong J, Chamberlain D, Wieczorek I, Fox KAA, Chesebro JH, Strain J, Keller C, Kelly A, Lancaster G, Ali J, Kronmal R, Fuster V and the Antithrombotic Therapy in Acute Coronary Syndromes Research Group: Combination antithrombotic therapy in unstable rest angina and non-Q wave infarction in nonprior aspirin users. Primary endpoints analysis from the ATACS trial. Circulation 1994;89:81–88.

7 Weitz JI: Low molecular weight heparins. N Engl J Med 1997;337:688–699.

8 Gurfinkel EP, Manos EJ, Mejail R, Cerda MA, Duronto EA, Garcia CN, Daroca AM, Mautner B: Low molecular weight heparin versus regular heparin in the treatment of unstable angina and silent ischaemia. J Am Coll Cardiol 1995;26: 313–318.

9 Wallentin L, Ohlsson J, Swahn E (for the FRISC Study Group): Low molecular weight heparin during instability in coronary artery disease. Lancet 1996;347:561–568.

10 Klein W, Buchwald A, Hillis SE, Monrad S, Sanz G, Turpie AGG, van der Meer J, Olaisson E, Undeland S, Ludwig K, for the FRIC Investigators: Comparison of low molecular weight heparin with unfractionated heparin acutely and with placebo for 6 weeks in the management of unstable coronary artery disease (FRIC). Circulation 1997; 96:61–68.

11 Cohen M, Demers C, Gurfinkel MD, Turpie AGG, Fromell GJ, Goodman S, Langer A, Califf RM, Fox KAA, Premmereur J, Bigonzi F, for the Efficacy and Safety of Subcutaneous Enoxaparin in Non-Q-Wave Coronary Events Study Group: A comparison of low molecular weight heparin with unfractionated heparin for unstable coronary artery disease. N Engl J Med 1997; 337:447–452.
12 Antman EM: The TIMI 11B Study. XXth Congress of the European Society of Cardiology, Vienna, Austria, August 25, 1998.
13 The FRAX.I.S Study Group: Comparison of two treatment durations (6 days and 14 days) of a low molecular weight heparin with a 6-day treatment of unfractionated heparin in the initial management of unstable angina or non-Q wave myocardial infarction: FRAX.I.S (FRAxiparine in Ischaemic Syndrome). Eur Heart J 1999;20:1553–1562.
14 The Fragmin During Instability in Coronary Artery Disease (FRISC II) Investigators: Invasive versus non-invasive strategy in unstable coronary artery disease – a prospective randomised multicentre study – the FRISC II invasive trial. Lancet 1999;354:708–715.
15 Mark DB, Cowper PA, Berkowitz SD, Davidson-Ray L, DeLong ER, Turpie AGG, Califf RM, Weatherley B, Cohen M: Economic assessment of low molecular weight heparin (enoxaparin) versus unfractionated heparin in acute coronary syndrome patients. Results from the ESSENCE randomized trial. Circulation 1998;97:1702–1707.
16 Cairns JA, Theroux P, Lewis HD, Ezekowitz M, Meade TW, Sutton GC: Antithrombotic agents in coronary artery disease. Chest 1998;114: S611–S633.

Workshop 1 Chairman: J.I. Weitz
New Antithrombotic Drugs: Beyond Aspirin and Heparin

Hæmostasis

Haemostasis 1999;29(suppl 1):76–78

Direct Thrombin Inhibitors

S. Anand

McMaster University, Hamilton General Hospital, Hamilton, Ont., Canada

Key Words
Acute coronary syndromes · Direct thrombin inhibitors · Hirudin · Bivalirudin

Abstract
Direct thrombin inhibitors may offer advantages over indirect thrombin inhibitors in the management of patients with acute coronary syndromes (ACS). Two direct thrombin inhibitors, hirudin and bivalirudin, have been investigated in Phase II and Phase III clinical trials. Based on the results of a meta-analysis of study data from 25,000 patients, hirudin appears to be more effective than unfractionated heparin (UFH) in the treatment of patients with ACS, but it is associated with an increased rate of major bleeding. A meta-analysis of a smaller patient population has suggested that bivalirudin, too, may be more efficacious than UFH and may also be safer.
Copyright © 1999 S. Karger AG, Basel

Acute coronary syndromes (ACS) represent a continuum of acute myocardial ischaemia, spanning from acute transmural infarction with ST segment elevation to unstable angina characterized by ischaemia without ST elevation. The current practice is to administer short-term antithrombotic therapy with intravenous heparin and aspirin in an effort to inhibit the development or extension of coronary thrombosis. Although this strategy is successful in the short term decreasing the incidence of cardiovascular events, in the long term, patients with ACS continue to have a high rate of recurrent ischaemic events.

Indirect thrombin inhibitors such as unfractionated heparin (UFH), although effective at inhibiting fluid-phase thrombin, are incapable of inhibiting clot-bound thrombin [1]. Clot-bound thrombin remains enzymatically active and is an intensely thrombogenic stimulus. There are theoretical advantages, therefore, in using direct thrombin inhibitors in patients with ACS. The direct thrombin

KARGER

Fax + 41 61 306 12 34
E-Mail karger@karger.ch
www.karger.com

© 1999 S. Karger AG, Basel
0301–0147/99/0297–0076$17.50/0

Accessible online at:
www.karger.com/journals/hae

Dr. S. Anand
Hamilton General Hospital
237 Barton Street East
Hamilton, Ont., L8L 2X2 (Canada)

inhibitors are able to inhibit the thrombin bound to fibrin and indirectly inhibit fluid-phase thrombin. Two direct thrombin inhibitors, hirudin and bivalirudin (formerly hirulog) have been subject to Phase II and Phase III clinical trials in the setting of ACS.

Hirudin is a 65-amino-acid protein derived from the saliva of the medicinal leech, and is now available in recombinant form. Recently, this agent, produced by Behringwerke AG, was tested in a large Phase III clinical trial involving 10,141 patients with ACS without ST elevation – OASIS-2 (Organization to Assess Strategies for Ischemic Syndromes-2) [2]. This was a randomized, double-blind controlled trial that directly compared hirudin (a bolus 0.4 mg/kg followed by 0.15 mg/kg/h) with UFH (a bolus 5,000 IU, and then 15 IU/kg/h). The activated partial thromboplastin time (APTT) was used to monitor both therapies, using a target range of 60 to 100 s. The primary pre-specified endpoint was a composite of cardiovascular (CV) death and recurrent myocardial infarction (MI) at 7 days. At 7 days, the event rate in the UFH group was 4.2% (214/5,058) compared with 3.6% (182/5,083) in the hirudin group, translating into approximately a 17% relative risk reduction in favour of hirudin ($p = 0.073$). In addition, a significant 18% risk reduction in revascularization procedures (including percutaneous transluminal coronary angioplasty and coronary artery bypass grafting) was also observed in patients who received hirudin. The absolute difference observed between the UFH and hirudin groups persisted at 35 days and at 180 days. The rate of major bleeding was 0.7% in patients treated with UFH, compared with 1.2% in patients treated with hirudin, resulting in a 1.71 times relative increase in bleeding with hirudin ($p = 0.01$). However, when this outcome was subdivided into life-threatening or non-life-threatening bleeds, no excess in life-threatening events occurred in the hirudin patients compared with the UFH patients.

A meta-analysis of study data from 25,000 patients with ACS who used hirudin with or without thrombolytic therapy indicates an absolute difference in CV death and MI between UFH and hirudin of 1%, which translates into a 16% reduction in hard CV endpoints, a result that is highly significant (OASIS Investigators, personal communication, 1999). Therefore, there is firm evidence that hirudin is more efficacious than UFH in treating patients with ACS.

Bivalirudin has potential theoretical benefits over hirudin. Unlike hirudin, which is slowly and reversibly bound to thrombin, bivalirudin is only transiently bound to the active site of thrombin. This means that it may still activate the endogenous protein C anticoagulation system, may allow larger doses of the agent to be given and offers the potential for increased efficacy and lower major bleeding complications. Bivalirudin is a semi-synthetic protein that is a much smaller compound than hirudin. A meta-analysis of previous trials using bivalirudin in arterial disease indicates an approximate 18% reduction in CV death and MI at 7 days with bivalirudin compared with UFH (S. Anand, unpublished results); the p value is not significant, however, as the confidence intervals around this estimate cross 1. Therefore, more data are needed to firmly delineate the efficacy of bivalirudin over UFH. Nevertheless, there are intriguing data to suggest that the rate of major bleeding may be significantly lower in patients treated with bivalirudin compared with those receiving UFH. In a meta-analysis incorporating many of the bivalirudin trials, a large risk reduction, in the order of 30–50%, is observed in patients treated with bivalirudin ($p < 0.0001$).

In summary, there are data from over 25,000 patients suggesting that hirudin is more efficacious than UFH in treating patients with ACS. However, it is also associated with an increased rate of major bleeding. There is preliminary evidence that bivalirudin is more efficacious than UFH; however, these are data from only approximately 5,000 patients, and more trial results are needed. Currently, the HERO-2 (Hirulog and Early Reperfusion/Occlusion-2) trial is planned in approximately 17,000 patients with acute MI, randomized to bivalirudin or UFH after thrombolytic therapy with streptokinase. The results of this trial will define the role of bivalirudin in the management of patients with ACS.

References

1 Weitz JI, Hudoba M, Massel D, Maraganore J, Hirsh J: Clot-bound thrombin is protected from inhibition by heparin-antithrombin III but is susceptible to inactivation by antithrombin III-independent inhibitors. J Clin Invest 1990;86:385–391.

2 Organisation to Assess Strategies for Ischemic Syndromes (OASIS-2) Investigators. Effects of recombinant hirudin (lepirudin) compared with heparin on death, myocardial infarction, refractory angina, and revascularisation procedures in patients with acute myocardial ischaemia without ST elevation: A randomised trial. Lancet 1999;353:429–438.

Hæmostasis

Haemostasis 1999;29(suppl 1):79–80

Optimization of Treatment for Venous Thromboembolism and Prevention of Recurrences

Co-Chairman's Summary

Sam Schulman Harry Büller

Coagulation Unit, Department of Haematology and Infectious Diseases, Karolinska Hospital, Stockholm, Sweden

The rationale for the use of thrombolytic therapy in venous thromboembolism (VTE) is to achieve rapid resolution of thrombin and improve the clinical outcome. In eight randomized clinical trials (RCTs) on deep vein thrombosis (DVT), thrombolytic therapy (streptokinase, SK, in six and tissue plasminogen activator, t-PA, in two) yielded marked resolution on venography in 48% of cases compared with 10% after unfractionated heparin (UFH). Unfortunately, there are no data on the benefit of thrombolytic therapy on the rate of recurrence and there are inconsistent data on its effect on the incidence of post-thrombotic syndrome. This is partly due to the low number of patients included in the eight studies – 144 in the heparin arms and 188 in the thrombolysis arms. The risk of major bleeding is 13.2 and 3.5% ($p < 0.004$) during treatment with thrombolytics and UFH, respectively.

The regimens that UFH has been compared with in pulmonary embolism (PE) are SK for 24 h, urokinase for 12 h and t-PA for 2 h. In five RCTs with a total of 368 patients, marked resolution after 24 h on perfusion scanning was seen in 8, 22 and 33% with UFH, SK and t-PA, respectively. However, after 14 days, the corresponding rates were 58–65, 52 and 53%, respectively. The rate of recurrence was 2–6, 2 and 7%, respectively. There are no data on the development of pulmonary hypertension, but the risk of major haemorrhage was 2–10, 4 and 17%, respectively. Patients with right ventricular dysfunction were shown to improve rapidly on thrombolytic therapy, and these should be studied in an RCT.

Although DVT is routinely treated with low-molecular-weight heparin (LMWH) at home in many countries, the RCTs excluded many subgroups. Patients with DVT extending as far proximally as into the iliac vein or with non-massive PE can receive this treatment. Previous thromboembolic episodes, or cancer, trauma or surgery as triggering causes do not contraindicate this choice. Some subgroups have not been studied, at least not in

KARGER

Fax +41 61 306 12 34
E-Mail karger@karger.ch
www.karger.com

© 1999 S. Karger AG, Basel

0301–0147/99/0297–0079$17.50/0

Accessible online at:
www.karger.com/journals/hae

Table 1. Recommendations for secondary prophylaxis after VTE

Location	Trigger	Duration	Evaluate
Distal DVT	Temporary	6 weeks	
Proximal DVT ± symptomatic PE	Temporary	3–6 months	3 vs. 6 months
Distal DVT	Permanent or idiopathic	6 months	Prolongation with low intensity
Proximal DVT	Permanent or idiopathic	6 months	Prolongation with low intensity
Any	+ Factor V Leiden heterozygous	as above	
Any	+ Factor II mutation heterozygous	as above	
Any	+ Cardiolipin antibodies	1 year then reassess	Full vs. low intensity
Any	+ Protein C/S deficiency heterozygous	6 months, then reassess	Full vs. low intensity
Any	+ Antithrombin deficiency	6 months, then reassess	
Any	+ Homocysteinaemia	6 months, then reassess	Folic acid and B12
Any	+ Combination/ homozygosity	1 year, then reassess or lifelong?	
Contralateral	Second VTE	As above	
Ipsilateral	Second VTE	At least 1 year	Prolongation with low intensity

RCTs. Older children should receive this mode of treatment. Pregnant patients should be studied. Increased bleeding risk, such as renal or liver failure, general illness, active haemorrhage or active peptic ulcer, precludes treatment as outpatients. Patients with renal failure should be studied with monitoring of anti-Xa levels in hospital and may then turn out to be manageable as outpatients. It is estimated that 85% of the patients with VTE can be treated with LMWH at home, thereby reducing the total cost by 50%. However, mobilization and compression therapy must not be neglected.

Based on available data from RCTs, recommendations were proposed for secondary prophylaxis after VTE, and these are outlined in table 1.

The prevalence of cancer has varied between 6 and 23% in VTE trials. For every 10% increase of cancer prevalence in a population, the risk of recurrence of VTE increases by 1.7% and the mortality rate per 3–6 months by 2.6%. Chemotherapy leads to a further increase of the risk of thromboembolic complications. Overall the RCTs assessing UFH versus LMWH (>4,000 patients), the odds ratio for 3-month mortality was 0.94 (95% CI, 0.6–1.5) in patients without cancer and 0.61 (0.4–0.93) in those with cancer. Thus, LMWH is the preferred treatment in VTE with cancer. In the secondary prophylaxis after VTE, LMWH is generally about equal to vitamin K antagonists but may be better in cancer patients. The duration of this prophylaxis should probably be longer in cancer patients than in those without cancer, but no solid data exist. The risk of major haemorrhage during secondary prophylaxis with vitamin K antagonists is higher in cancer patients (13 versus 2% annually), but the risk of thromboembolic events is also much higher (28 versus 8%). There is no proven benefit of vena caval filters in cancer patients.

Workshop 2 Chairmen: H. Büller, S. Schulman
Optimization of Treatment for VTE and Prevention of Recurrences

Hæmostasis

Haemostasis 1999;29(suppl 1):81–83

Is There a Role for Thrombolytic Therapy in Venous Thromboembolism?

Bernd-Jan Sanson Harry Büller

Department of Vascular Medicine, Academic Medical Centre, Amsterdam, The Netherlands

Key Words
Thrombolytic therapy · Deep vein thrombosis · Pulmonary embolism

Abstract
Theoretically, thrombolytic therapy would appear to offer benefits over standard heparin therapy in the treatment of venous thromboembolism based on the more rapid resolution of thrombus. In this paper, the results of clinical trials performed with thrombolytic agents in the initial treatment of both deep vein thrombosis (DVT) and pulmonary embolism (PE) are reviewed. Although there have been positive findings with surrogate markers, studies to date have failed to demonstrate that thrombolytic therapy is associated with an improved long-term clinical outcome in patients with DVT or PE. Recent reports have suggested that thrombolytic agents could be clinically useful in a subgroup who have right ventricular dysfunction on echocardiography. Randomized clinical trials, with clinically relevant endpoints, are required to determine the efficacy and safety of thrombolytic therapy in these patients.

Copyright © 1999 S. Karger AG, Basel

Introduction

The role of thrombolytic therapy in the treatment of patients with venous thromboembolism (VTE) remains questionable despite many years of research in this field. Thrombolytic therapy has been suggested by some for the initial treatment of both acute deep vein thrombosis (DVT) and pulmonary embolism (PE). The rationale for the use of thrombolytic therapy is based on the potentially more rapid resolution of thrombi with such therapy than with standard heparin treatment alone.

KARGER

Fax + 41 61 306 12 34
E-Mail karger@karger.ch
www.karger.com

© 1999 S. Karger AG, Basel
0301–0147/99/0297–0081$17.50/0

Accessible online at:
www.karger.com/journals/hae

Dr. B.J. Sanson
Department of Vascular Medicine
Academic Medical Centre
Meibergdreef 9
1105 AZ, Amsterdam (The Netherlands)

Theoretically, in the treatment of DVT, the potential benefit of thrombolytic therapy could lie in the following aspects:

- Direct resolution of an obstructive thrombus may be associated with quicker relief of the accompanying symptoms.
- Rapid resolution of the thrombus may be associated with less extensive valve damage and, as such, could result in a decrease in long-term complications such as the post-thrombotic syndrome.
- More complete resolution of the thrombus could lead to a lower incidence of recurrent VTE.

Similarly, in the treatment of PE, the potential benefit could theoretically lie in the following aspects:

- Thrombolysis could lead to a rapid restitution of lung perfusion, with potential short-term clinical benefit.
- A decrease in the vascular resistance could reduce the long-term development of right ventricular heart dysfunction and pulmonary hypertension.
- Based on the assumption that the source for PE is more completely resolved, there could be a lower incidence of recurrent VTE.

Deep Vein Thrombosis

There have been eight properly performed, randomized, controlled studies comparing thrombolytic therapy and unfractionated heparin (UFH) in the initial treatment of DVT [1]. Streptokinase was used in six of these studies and recombinant tissue plasminogen activator (rt-PA) was used in the remaining two. A total of 144 patients were included in the UFH arms, whereas 188 patients received thrombolytic therapy. All studies demonstrated a statistically significant reduction of thrombus size in favour of thrombolytic therapy, with moderate to significant thrombolysis being achieved 2.9 times more often in patients treated with thrombolytics than in those receiving UFH. Major bleeding, requiring medical attention, was observed in 13.2% of patients treated with thrombolytic agents and in 3.5% of patients treated with UFH (relative increase of 3.8; $p < 0.004$). Large studies, with long-term follow-up, evaluating the development of the post-thrombotic syndrome in patients treated with thrombolytic therapy versus standard heparin therapy are lacking, although small studies have revealed both advantageous and deleterious effects [2, 3]. Furthermore, there are no clinical data showing a reduction in the risk of recurrent VTE after thrombolysis.

Table 1. Perfusion-scan resolution in studies comparing thrombolytic therapy and UFH in patients with PE

	24 h	5–7 days	14 days
UPET			
Urokinase	22%	41%	52%
UFH	8%	36%	58%
rt-PA trials			
rt-PA	33%	51%	53%
UFH	8%	44%	65%

UPET = Urokinase in Pulmonary Embolism Trial.

Pulmonary Embolism

There have been several randomized controlled trials comparing the use of thrombolytic agents with UFH in the treatment of patients with PE. The single largest study, the UPET (Urokinase in Pulmonary Embolism Trial), performed in 1973, included 160 patients [4], whereas four rt-PA studies included a total of 208 patients [5–8]. In these studies, thrombolytic therapy was associated with a significant improvement of lung perfusion, as assessed by scintigraphy, within the first day of treatment, although a lasting benefit on perfusion was not apparent during subsequent days of follow-up (table 1). Significant differences in the decrease of mean pulmonary artery pressure after 2 h of treatment, in favour of thrombolytic therapy, have been reported. Despite these positive findings with surrogate markers, these studies have not shown a significant improvement in the long-term clinical outcome of patients treated with thrombolytic agents – the incidences of recurrent VTE and mortality were not decreased, while the incidence of major bleeding was significantly higher in patients treated with thrombolytics.

Conclusion

Although thrombolytic therapy would appear to offer theoretical advantages over standard treatment with UFH for DVT and PE, no studies have unequivocally demonstrated that the long-term clinical outcome is indeed improved. Consequently, thrombolytic therapy is not considered to be routinely indicated in such patients. However, recent reports have suggested that thrombolytic agents could be clinically useful in a subgroup of haemodynamically stable patients with PE who have right ventricular dysfunction, as revealed by echocardiography, which has been shown to be associated with an increased risk of mortality [9]. Randomized clinical trials, with clinically relevant outcome measures, evaluating the efficacy and safety of thrombolytic therapy in these patients are needed.

References

1 Hirsh J, Salzman EW, Marder VJ: Treatment of venous thromboembolism; in Colman RW, Hirsh J, Marder VJ, Salzman EW (eds): Hemostasis and Thrombosis, Basic Principles and Clinical Practice, ed 3. Philadelphia, Lippincott, 1994, pp. 1346–1366.

2 Elliot MS, Immelman EJ, Jeffery P, Benatar SR, Funston MR, Smith JA, Shepstone BJ, Ferguson AD, Jacobs P, Walker W, Louw JH: A comparative randomized trial of heparin versus streptokinase in the treatment of acute proximal venous thrombosis: An interim report of a prospective trial. Br J Surg 1979;66: 838–843.

3 Kakkar VV, Lawrence D: Hemodynamic and clinical assessment after therapy for acute deep vein thrombosis: A prospective study. Am J Surg 1985;150:54–63.

4 The Urokinase Pulmonary Embolism Trial: A national cooperative study. Circulation 1973;47(suppl 2): 1–108.

5 PIOPED Investigators: Tissue plasminogen activator for the treatment of acute pulmonary embolism. Chest 1990;97:528–533.

6 Levine M, Hirsh J, Weitz J, Cruickshank M, Neemeh J, Turpie AG, Gent M: A randomized trial of a single bolus dosage regimen of recombinant tissue plasminogen activator in patients with acute pulmonary embolism. Chest 1990;98:1473–1479.

7 Dalla-Volta S, Palla A, Santolicandro A, Giuntini C, Pengo V, Visioli O, Zonzin P, Zanuttini D, Barbaresi F, Agnelli G: PAIMS 2 – Alteplase combined with heparin versus heparin in the treatment of acute pulmonary embolism: Plasminogen Activator Italian Multicenter Study 2. J Am Coll Cardiol 1992;20:250–226.

8 Goldhaber SZ, Haire WD, Feildstein ML, Miller M, Toltzis R, Smith JL, Taveria da Silva AM, Come PC, Lee RT, Parker JA: Alteplase versus heparin in acute pulmonary embolism: Randomized trial assessing right ventricular function and pulmonary perfusion. Lancet 1993;341:507–511.

9 Goldhaber SZ, Visani L, De Rosa M, for ICOPER: Acute pulmonary embolism: Clinical outcomes in the International Cooperative Pulmonary Embolism Registry (ICOPER). Lancet 1999;353:1386–1389.

Workshop 2 Chairmen: H. Büller, S. Schulman
Optimization of Treatment for Venous Thromboembolism and Prevention of Recurrences

Hæmostasis

Haemostasis 1999;29(suppl 1):84–88

Can All Patients with Deep Vein Thrombosis Receive Low-Molecular-Weight Heparin in an Outpatient Setting?

Per Lindmarker

Coagulation Unit, Division of Haematology, Karolinska Hospital, Stockholm, Sweden

Key Words

Low-molecular-weight heparin · Outpatient · Venous thromboembolism · Feasibility

Abstract

Studies have shown subcutaneous low-molecular-weight heparin (LMWH) to be at least as safe and efficacious as intravenous unfractionated heparin (UFH) for the treatment of venous thromboembolism (VTE). Furthermore, unlike UFH, LMWH is administered on a once- or twice-daily basis without monitoring in uncomplicated cases. Consequently, it has been suggested that the large majority of patients with VTE could be treated on an outpatient basis. Exceptions include patients with an increased risk of haemorrhage, pregnant women, children and those with renal insufficiency. Outpatient management would offer economic advantages and be more convenient for both the patient and the hospital staff.

Copyright © 1999 S. Karger AG, Basel

In the past decade, trials have been performed comparing continuous intravenous unfractionated heparin (UFH) with low-molecular-weight heparins (LMWHs), administered subcutaneously, once or twice daily, in doses adjusted for body weight, for treatment of venous thromboembolism (VTE). The frequencies of bleeding and recurrent VTE have been very consistent despite the use of different LMWHs, whereas the results in UFH-treated patients have varied considerably from one trial to another [1–7]. There is convincing evidence that LMWHs are at least as safe and effective as UFH in the initial treatment of acute deep vein thrombosis (DVT) and probably also for pulmonary embolism [8].

From these results emerged the possibility for a shift towards treatment of VTE in an outpatient setting. A previous pilot study of outpatient treatment had shown encouraging results [9]. This strategy allows for substantial cost-savings to be made in comparison with traditional in-hospital care and is more convenient for the patients and hospital staff.

KARGER

Fax + 41 61 306 12 34
E-Mail karger@karger.ch
www.karger.com

© 1999 S. Karger AG, Basel
0301–0147/99/0297–0084$17.50/0

Accessible online at:
www.karger.com/journals/hae

Dr. P. Lindmarker
Coagulation Unit, Division of Haematology
Karolinska Hospital
SE–171 76 Stockholm (Sweden)

Table 1. Summary of results in four studies [10–13] investigating treatment of DVT with LMWH in an outpatient setting

	Lindmarker et al. (1996) [10]	Levine et al. (1996) [11]		Koopman et al. (1996) [12]		Columbus (1997) [13]	
Randomized controlled trial	No	Yes		Yes		Yes	
LMWH compound	Dalteparin	Enoxaparin		Nadroparin		Reviparin	
Dose administered subcutaneously	200 IU/kg × 1	1 mg/kg × 2		4,100, 6,150 or 9,200 IU × 2		3,500, 4,200 or 6,300 IU × 2	
Patients receiving LMWH	434	247		202		510	
Treated as outpatients only	152 (35%)	120 (49%)		72 (36%)		100 (20%)	
Treated as inpatients <48 h	85 (20%)	≈60 (24%)		44 (22%)		56 (11%)	
Endpoints	LMWH	LMWH	UFH	LMWH	UFH	LMWH	UFH
Recurrent VTE within 3 months	1.6%	5.3%	6.7%	6.9%	8.6%	5.3%	4.9%
Major bleeding (initial period)	0.2%[1]	2.0%[2]	1.2%[2]	1.0%[3]	0.55%[3]	2.0%[3]	1.6%[3]
		n.s.		n.s.		n.s.	

During initial treatment +72 h[1] or +48 h[2]; 0–14 days[3].

Table 2. Summary of patient characteristics in four studies [10–13] investigating treatment of DVT with LMWH in an outpatient setting

Included	Lindmarker et al. (1996)	Levine et al. (1996)	Koopman et al. (1996)	Columbus (1997)
Distal DVT	Yes	No	No	Yes
Proximal DVT	Yes	Yes	Yes	Yes
Malignancy (%)	5.1	19	18	23
Surgery ≤3 months (%)	11.3	21	16	32
Trauma ≤3 months (%)	ND	8	11	11
Previous VTE (%)	ND	21	19	20

ND = no data.

Recent studies have compared the tolerability and efficacy of four different LMWHs administered in an outpatient setting with intravenous UFH administered in hospital [10–13]. The results regarding recurrent VTE episodes, major bleeding and death were similar in the LMWH and UFH groups, as shown in tables 1 and 2. In a non-randomized multicentre feasibility study of LMWH conducted among 434 patients, the frequency of recurrent VTE during the LMWH treatment and the entire 3-month study period was 0.7 and 1.6%, respectively [13].

In all these trials, including 1,393 patients on LMWH, there has been a selection of patients. Not all eligible patients have been

Table 3. Summary of exclusion criteria in four studies [10–13] investigating treatment of DVT with LMWH in an outpatient setting

Exclusion criteria	Lindmarker et al. (1996)	Levine et al. (1996)	Koopman et al. (1996)	Columbus (1997)
Age < 18 years	X		X	X
Inability for outpatient treatment		X		
Symptomatic pulmonary embolism	X	X	X	No (27%)
Pregnancy and nursing	X	X	X	X
Life expectancy < 6 months			X	
Coagulation inhibitor deficiency		X		
Previous VTE episodes		≥2	≤2 years	
Post-thrombotic syndrome			X	
Major surgery	≤15 days			≤3 days
Thrombocytopenia (< 100,000 mm^3)	X			X
Familial bleeding disorder	X	X		
Currently active bleeding	X	X		X
Active peptic ulcer disease	X	X		X
Hepatic insufficiency	X			
Renal insufficiency	X			

Table 4. Subjective interpretation of accumulated data and experience up to date regarding whether certain subgroups of patients with DVT are suitable or not for outpatient treatment

Subgroup of patient	Outpatient treatment accurate?
Age < 18 years	?No (insufficient data)
Pregnancy and nursing	?No (insufficient data)
Increased risk of recurrent VTE	
Previous VTE episodes	Yes
Malignant disease	Yes
Symptomatic pulmonary embolism	Probably in uncomplicated cases (insufficient data)
Post-thrombotic syndrome	Yes
Increased risk of bleeding	
Bleeding tendency disorder	No
Renal insufficiency	Only in selected cases and anti-Factor Xa monitoring available
Hepatic insufficiency	No
Recent surgery	No
Currently active bleeding	No
Active peptic ulcer disease	No

included (table 3). However, the data available are convincing that most patients with DVT or non-massive pulmonary embolism, and without concomitant disease or additional risk factors for recurrent VTE and bleeding, can be treated as outpatients with LMWH [1–13].

Which patients are not suitable for outpatient regimens? There is no documentation available for certain patient groups and in others it is insufficient. We have no trials for individuals aged less than 18 years, pregnant women or for patients with an increased bleeding risk. Interpretations have to be made concerning suitable patients for outpatient treatment not included in the trials, and we have no data to support a general recommendation for outpatient treatment of all VTE patients. Patients with previous VTE, post-thrombotic syndrome or coagulation inhibitor deficiencies can probably be treated as outpatients. Compared with non-cancer patients, the risk of recurrent VTE was doubled in patients with malignant disease, in both the LMWH and UFH groups, but an outpatient regimen seems justified [10]. It appears that patients with an increased bleeding risk – such as recent surgery or trauma, impaired haemostasis or currently active bleeding – should be treated in hospital and not as outpatients. For patients with renal insufficiency, in-hospital treatment is probably more accurate. The feasibility of treating a large majority (>80%) of VTE patients as outpatients has been confirmed in other studies [14, 15]. This strategy allows for substantial cost-savings to be made in comparison with traditional in-hospital care [16].

Conclusions

In conclusion, although not all, the vast majority of patients with DVT, and probably also some with non-massive pulmonary embolism, can be treated with LMWH in an outpatient setting without impairment of safety and efficacy (table 4).

References

1 Hull RD, Raskob GE, Pineo GF, Green D, Trowbridge AA, Elliott CG, Lerner RG, Hall J, Sparling T, Brettell HR: Subcutaneous low-molecular-weight heparin compared with continuous intravenous heparin in the treatment of proximal-vein thrombosis. N Engl J Med 1992;326:975–982.
2 Prandoni P, Lensing AWA, Buller HR, Carta M, Cogo A, Vigo M, Casara D, Ruol A, ten Cate JW: Comparison of subcutaneous low-molecular-weight heparin with intravenous standard heparin in proximal deep-vein thrombosis. Lancet 1992; 339:441–445.
3 Lindmarker P, Holmstrom M, Granqvist S, Johnson H, Lockneer D: Comparison of once-daily subcutaneous Fragmin with continuous intravenous unfractionated heparin in the treatment of deep vein thrombosis. Thromb Haemost 1994;72: 186–190.
4 Lopaciuk S, Meissner A, Filipecki S, Zawilska K, Sowier J, Ciesielski L, Bielawiec M, Glowinski S, Czestochowska E: Subcutaneous low molecular weight heparin versus subcutaneous unfractionated heparin in the treatment of deep vein thrombosis: A Polish multicenter trial. Thromb Haemost 1992;68:14–18.
5 Luomanmaki K, Grankvist S, Hallert C, Jauro I, Ketola K, Kim HC, Kiviniemi H, Koskivirta H, Sorskog L, Vikko P: A multicentre comparison of once-daily subcutaneous dalteparin (low molecular weight heparin) and continuous intravenous heparin in the treatment of deep vein thrombosis. J Intern Med 1996; 240:85–92.
6 Fiessinger JN, Lopez-Fernandez M, Gatterer E, Granqvist S, Kher A, Olsson CG: Once-daily subcutaneous dalteparin, a low molecular weight heparin, for the initial treatment of acute deep vein thrombosis. Thromb Haemost 1996;76:195–199.
7 Duroux P, Beelere A: A randomised trial of subcutaneous low molecular weight heparin (CY 216) compared with intravenous unfractionated heparin in the treatment of deep vein thrombosis. A collaborative European multicentre study. Thromb Haemost 1991;65:251–256.

8 Simonneau G, Sors H, Charbonnier B, Page Y, Laaban JP, Azarian R, Laurent M, Hirsch JL, Ferrari E, Bosson JL, Mottier D, Beau B: A comparison of low-molecular-weight heparin with unfractionated heparin for acute pulmonary embolism. N Engl J Med 1997;337:663–669.
9 Blattler W: Ambulatory care for ambulant patients with deep vein thrombosis. J Mal Vasculaires 1991; 16:137–141.
10 Lindmarker P, Holmstrom M: Use of low molecular weight heparin (dalteparin), once daily, for the treatment of deep vein thrombosis. A feasibility and health economic study in an outpatient setting. Swedish Venous Thrombosis Dalteparin Trial Group. J Intern Med 1996; 240:395–401.
11 Levine M, Gent M, Hirsh J, Leclerc J, Anderson D, Weitz J, Ginsberg J, Turpie AGG, Demers C, Kovacs M: A comparison of low-molecular-weight heparin administered primarily at home with unfractionated heparin administered in the hospital for proximal deep-vein thrombosis. N Engl J Med 1996;334:677–681.
12 Koopman MM, Prandoni P, Piovella F, Ockleford PA, Brandjes DPM, van der Meer J, Gallus AS, Simonneau G, Chesterman CH, Prins MH, Bossuyt PMM, de Haes H, van den Belt AGM, Sagnard L, d'Azemar P, Buller HR: Treatment of venous thrombosis with intravenous unfractionated heparin administered in the hospital as compared with subcutaneous low-molecular-weight heparin administered at home. The TASMAN Study Group. N Engl J Med 1996;334:682–687.
13 The Columbus Investigators: Low-molecular-weight heparin in the treatment of patients with venous thromboembolism. N Engl J Med 1997;337:657–662.
14 Wells PS, Kovacs MJ, Bormanis J, Forgie MA, Goudie D, Morrow B, Kovacs J: Expanding eligibility for outpatient treatment of deep vein thrombosis and pulmonary embolism with low-molecular-weight heparin: A comparison of patient self-injection with homecare injection. Arch Intern Med 1998;158:1809–1812.
15 Grau E, Real E, Pastor E, Viciano V, Aguilo J: Home treatment of deep vein thrombosis: A two-year experience of a single institution. Haematologica 1998;83:438–441.
16 van den Belt AG, Bossuyt PM, Prins MH, Gallus AS, Buller HR: Replacing inpatient care by outpatient care in the treatment of deep venous thrombosis – an economic evaluation. TASMAN Study Group. Thromb Haemost 1998;79:259–263.

Workshop 2 Chairmen: H. Büller, S. Schulman
Optimization of Treatment for Venous Thromboembolism and Prevention of Recurrences

Hæmostasis

Haemostasis 1999;29(suppl 1):89–90

For How Long Should the Treatment with Vitamin K Antagonists Be Maintained?

Sam Schulman

Coagulation Unit, Department of Haematology and Infectious Disease, Karolinska Hospital, Stockholm, Sweden

Key Words
Vitamin K antagonists · Thromboprophylaxis · Venous thromboembolism

Abstract
Studies have shown that in most patients with venous thromboembolism (VTE), continuation of treatment with vitamin K antagonists for up to 27 months significantly reduces the probability of recurrence. Likewise, prolongation of oral anticoagulation beyond 6 months is believed to be of benefit in patients with certain forms of hereditary thrombophilia. Very prolonged periods of treatment with vitamin K antagonists at standard doses, although conferring benefit regarding the risk of recurrence of VTE, are associated with an increased incidence of major bleeds and require intensive monitoring. Use of a lower intensity of anticoagulation may reduce these negative aspects and enable anticoagulation to be carried out for longer.

Copyright © 1999 S. Karger AG, Basel

Introduction

Recent prospective randomized studies on the optimal duration of oral anticoagulation with vitamin K antagonists after venous thromboembolism (VTE) have demonstrated that the probability of recurrence is reduced when the secondary prophylaxis is prolonged from 4 weeks to 3 months [1] or from 6 weeks to 6 months [6] or from 3 months to 27 months [3]. The patient material and the duration of follow-up differed, however, between these trials.

KARGER

Fax + 41 61 306 12 34
E-Mail karger@karger.ch
www.karger.com

© 1999 S. Karger AG, Basel
0301–0147/99/0297–0089$17.50/0

Accessible online at:
www.karger.com/journals/hae

Dr. S. Schulman
Coagulation Unit
Department of Haematology and Infectious Diseases
Karolinska Hospital
SE–171 76 Stockholm (Sweden)

Treatment Recommendations

The reduced risk of recurrence is valid for patients except those with the combination of a calf vein thrombosis and a temporary triggering risk factor, such as surgery. For this subgroup of patients, a prolongation of secondary prophylaxis beyond 6 weeks is not of any benefit. In patients with proximal deep vein thrombosis (DVT) or symptomatic pulmonary embolism (SPE) and a temporary trigger, a prolongation from 6 weeks to 6 months yields a significantly lower incidence of recurrence; however, this difference is not significant after 3–4 years, and the optimal duration may be between 3 and 6 months. For those with an idiopathic or permanent triggering factor and any DVT or SPE, a prolongation from 6 weeks to 6 months confers a significant advantage regarding the incidence of recurrence, which remains even after 6 years. Even longer durations should be considered in patients with cardiolipin antibodies, because of a significantly higher probability of recurrence and a higher mortality caused by all kinds of thrombotic events after cessation of anticoagulation at 6 months [4]. The risk of recurrence is of the same magnitude in patients with proximal DVT or with SPE.

Patients with hereditary thrombophilia caused by a heterozygous mutation of factor V Leiden or prothrombin do not seem to run an increased risk of recurrence [5]. For the heterozygous forms of protein C, protein S or antithrombin deficiency, the risk of recurrence is at least 10% per year [6], which is twice that in patients without hereditary thrombophilia, and a prolongation beyond 6 months is warranted. Patients with hyperhomocysteinaemia also are at an increased risk of recurrence, but substitution with folate [7] and vitamin B12 [8] may provide a better benefit/risk ratio than vitamin K antagonists.

After the second event of VTE, prolongation of oral anticoagulation from 6 months to 48 months markedly reduces the rate of recurrence, but with a trend towards more major haemorrhages in the latter group [9]. Other arguments against very long durations of conventional treatment with vitamin K antagonists, aiming at an international normalized ratio (INR) of 2.0–3.0, are the necessity of monitoring the prothrombin time, which has direct and indirect costs, and the constant fear of interactions with other drugs and food products. These have to be weighed against the reduction or elimination of a risk of recurrence of about 5% per year after cessation of anticoagulation.

Conclusions

If a lower intensity of anticoagulation (INR 1.5–2.0) turns out to be safer and more convenient – i.e. is associated with a lower incidence of bleeding complications and allows for less frequent monitoring of prothrombin time – the recommendations for the duration of anticoagulation will require revision.

Workshop 2 Chairmen: H. Büller, S. Schulman
Optimization of Treatment for Venous Thromboembolism and Prevention of Recurrences

Haemostasis

Haemostasis 1999;29(suppl 1):91–97

Should Patients with Venous Thromboembolism and Cancer Be Treated Differently?

Susanne M. Smorenburg[a] Barbara A. Hutten[b] Martin H. Prins[b]

[a]Department of Vascular Medicine and Cell Biology and Histology, Academic Medical Centre, [b]Department of Clinical Epidemiology and Biostatistics, University of Amsterdam, Amsterdam, The Netherlands

Key Words
Venous thromboembolism · Cancer · Vitamin K antagonists · Low-molecular-weight heparin · Recurrent venous thromboembolism · Bleeding

Abstract
Patients with malignant disease constitute a significant subgroup among patients with venous thromboembolism. Current results suggest that cancer patients are not only at an increased risk for thromboembolic events, particularly during chemotherapy treatment or after surgery, they also have an increased risk for bleeding complications while receiving oral anticoagulant treatment. The exact incidences of venous thromboembolic complications for the various types of cancer, however, are not well determined. Recent studies have indicated that subcutaneous low-molecular-weight heparin (LMWH) is as safe and effective as intravenous unfractionated heparin (UFH) in the initial treatment of venous thromboembolism. Moreover, a meta-analysis has provided preliminary evidence that, compared with UFH, LMWH treatment may prolong survival in cancer patients. Initiation of LMWH treatment in these patients is, therefore, recommended. Prospective randomized clinical trials to assess the optimum dose and duration of therapy are called for.

Copyright © 1999 S. Karger AG, Basel

Introduction

Patients with active cancer represent an important subgroup among patients with venous thromboembolism (VTE). Several, sometimes conflicting, reports have been published on the relation of the presence of malignancy and the risk of both recurrent venous

KARGER
Fax + 41 61 306 12 34
E-Mail karger@karger.ch
www.karger.com

© 1999 S. Karger AG, Basel
0301–0147/99/0297–0091$17.50/0

Accessible online at:
www.karger.com/journals/hae

Dr. M.H. Prins
Department of Clinical Epidemiology and Biostatistics
Room J2–228, Academic Medical Centre
University of Amsterdam, PO Box 22700
1100 DE Amsterdam (The Netherlands)

thromboembolic and bleeding complications among patients with VTE. If rates of these complications are indeed higher among patients with malignancy, this could have an influence on both the therapeutic approach in cancer patients with VTE and the design of trials that are intended to optimize the treatment of venous thrombosis in these patients. In this review, we firstly try to assess the numerical importance of the subgroup of patients with malignancy and VTE. Thereafter, the differences in complication rates and their potential consequences for both initial and long-term treatment phases are reviewed.

Prevalence of Malignancy among Patients with VTE

It is commonly assumed that the risk of thromboembolic complications is increased in patients with active cancer. Clinically overt thromboembolic complications have been observed in up to 26% of patients with cancer, whereas considerably higher incidences of thrombosis, up to 50%, have been observed in post mortem studies, especially in patients with mucinous carcinomas of the lung, pancreas and gastrointestinal tract [1–3].

The enhanced risk of thrombosis in patients with cancer can partly be explained by disturbances in the haemostatic and fibrinolytic system [4]. Indeed, laboratory evidence of intravascular coagulation and/or fibrinolytic activation can be detected in almost all cancer patients [5]. However, there is no clear association between changes in laboratory clotting or fibrinolytic indicators and the occurrence of subsequently clinically manifest thrombosis [1, 6]. In addition to the enhanced risk of venous thrombosis caused by the tumour, comorbid predisposing factors such as immobility, surgery, the use of central venous catheters and chemotherapeutic agents can enhance the risk of venous thromboembolic complications. For most types of cancer, there is a lack of prospective studies documenting the precise incidence of thromboembolic complications.

Reliable information on the incidence of thromboembolism with and without anticancer treatment is available for patients with breast cancer. In the absence of treatment, the incidence of VTE in patients with stage I and II breast cancer is comparable with that in the general population (approximately 0.2% in 4 years) [7–9]. Higher incidences have been observed in patients who receive chemotherapy, especially in women who are postmenopausal [10–14]. The combination of chemotherapy and hormonal treatment further enhances the risk of thromboembolic complications (incidences of 2.8 to 8.0% during 6–12 months of treatment). These trials thus suggest that anticancer treatment, especially combined hormonal therapy and chemotherapy, significantly contributes to venous thrombosis in patients with early stages of breast cancer. In patients with metastatic breast cancer, equivalent or higher incidences of thromboembolic complications have been observed during approximately 6 months of chemotherapeutic treatment (4.4–8.2%) [15, 16]. The incidence figures, however, might be influenced by the times of observation.

The incidence of thrombotic complications during chemotherapeutic treatment has also been investigated in patients with high-grade gliomas. In a prospective study, the incidence of clinically overt deep vein thrombosis (DVT) among 77 patients receiving adjuvant chemotherapy following surgery for high-grade gliomas was 26% (n = 20) during a follow-up period of 74.4 weeks [17]. Four of these 20 patients had massive pulmonary embolism. The highest incidence was found in the first 7 months after surgery, when chemotherapy was still being administered. In a ret-

Table 1. Distribution of types of malignancy in three recent clinical trials which compared LMWH to UFH for the initial treatment of VTE [23]

Primary site of malignancy at entry	Number of patients (%)	Number of deaths at 3 months (%)
Genitourinary tract	118 (29%)	13 (11%)
Gastrointestinal tract	80 (20%)	24 (30%)
Breast	57 (14%)	3 (5%)
Respiratory	42 (10%)	20 (48%)
Haematological	40 (10%)	4 (10%)
Central nervous system	37 (9%)	10 (27%)
Other	31 (8%)	3 (10%)
Total	405 (100%)	77 (19%)

rospective analysis of 77 patients with high-grade gliomas, 15 patients (19%) had clinically manifest DVT or pulmonary embolism during the course of their disease [18]. Twelve of these patients were receiving chemotherapy when thrombosis occurred. In contrast, the incidence of clinically manifest venous thrombosis or embolism among 1,703 patients who underwent initial craniotomy for gliomas, meningiomas or cerebral metastasis was 1.6% within 4 weeks of surgery [19]. None of these patients received chemotherapy. Although the results of this last and the two other studies might seem dissimilar, the differences can be entirely explained by variation in the duration of follow-up. Higher incidences of thromboses following surgery for various types of malignancies have been reported. However, in most of these studies, the presence of DVT was detected by fibrinogen leg scan; thus, many of these thrombi were, in fact, asymptomatic [20, 21].

Although the precise risk of thrombosis in cancer patients is unknown, these patients represent a significant subgroup of all patients with VTE. In randomized trials that compared low-molecular-weight heparin (LMWH) with unfractionated heparin (UFH) for the initial treatment of symptomatic VTE, the proportion of cancer patients included varied between 6 and 23%, with a mean prevalence of 16% [22]. The distribution of specific types of malignancies was available for three trials, including a total of 405 cancer patients (table 1) [23]. The prevalence of the various malignancies in these trials seemed to follow the frequency of cancer in the general population. Thus, since patients with cancer have an enhanced risk of thrombosis, the prevalence of cancer patients among all patients with venous thromboembolic complications is high.

Complications During the Treatment Period

Patients with confirmed VTE are usually initially treated with UFH or LMWH for at least 5 days. Treatment with vitamin K antagonists is started concomitantly and continued for at least 3 months. This strategy is similar for patients with and without concomitant malignant disease.

A recent meta-analysis of all published randomized clinical trials comparing UFH with LMWH for the initial treatment of VTE observed a non-significant decrease in the rate of recurrent VTE associated with LMWH use [3.8 vs. 4.8%; common odds ratio (OR)

0.77; 95% CI, 0.56–1.04], a significant decrease in the risk of major bleeds (1.3 vs. 2.2%; OR 0.60; 95% CI, 0.38–0.95) and a significant decrease in the 3-month mortality rate (4.8 vs. 6.5%; OR 0.72; 95% CI, 0.55–0.96) [22]. It can therefore be concluded that LMWHs were at least as efficacious as, but safer than, UFH. Interestingly, the patients with malignancy included in the individual trials had a statistically significant influence on both the incidence of recurrent thromboembolic events and the mortality observed in these trials. A 10% increase in the proportion of patients with malignancy increased the incidence of recurrent VTE by 1.7% (95% CI, 0.1–3.2%) and that of mortality by 2.6% (95% CI, 1.1–4.1%) [22]. In addition, it has been demonstrated that the decreased mortality among patients treated with LMWH can entirely be explained by the decreased mortality among patients with cancer [22, 24]. Consequently, the initial use of LMWH can be strongly recommended for patients presenting with VTE who have an underlying malignancy. Also, it can be concluded that this subgroup significantly affects outcome rates in clinical trials evaluating antithrombotic agents. Therefore, the proportion of patients with cancer in each study should be taken into account when comparing results from individual studies.

The situation with regard to the preferred long-term treatment in patients with cancer is less clear. In a recent cohort study it was shown that patients with malignancy are not only at higher risk for thromboembolic events than patients without malignancy (28 vs. 8% annually), but also have an increased risk for haemorrhagic complications while receiving treatment with vitamin K antagonists (13 vs. 2% annually) [25]. Similar results were obtained by Bona et al. [26], although the differences did not reach statistical significance due to the low number of patients included in their study. Prandoni [27] found an increased risk for recurrent VTE, but a similar risk for major bleeding, in cancer patients as compared with non-cancer patients. Moreover, Bona et al. [26] reported that patients with malignant disease spent more time outside the therapeutic range of the international normalized ratio (INR), despite more frequent monitoring. These findings suggest that treatment with vitamin K antagonists could be improved or alternative treatments should be considered. A possible alternative to oral anticoagulants in the prevention of recurrences is LMWH. Three recent randomized studies have evaluated the long-term use of LMWHs compared with vitamin K antagonists in the secondary prophylaxis of VTE [28–30]. The incidences of recurrent VTE and major bleeding were similar in patients treated with LMWHs as compared with those who received vitamin K antagonists, while the incidence of minor bleeding complications was significantly lower among the LMWH recipients. In a large cohort study, a similar reduction of major bleeding during long-term treatment with LMWH was observed [31]. Trials with prolonged LMWH therapy, focussing specifically on patients with VTE and underlying cancer, are not currently available. Since in the above-mentioned trials the dosage of LMWH used was lower than that recommended for initial treatment, it is conceivable that with the long-term use of therapeutic dosages a better protection against recurrences could be obtained, albeit at a price of a bleeding rate similar to that seen with vitamin K antagonists.

Classically, the duration of oral anticoagulant treatment is 3–6 months in most patients. Recent evidence, however, suggests that prolongation of vitamin K antagonists beyond this period may be beneficial among patients at high risk of recurrence. Because patients with active malignancy are reported to be at a particularly high risk of recurrent VTE, it is likely, although not documented, that prolongation of treatment is also beneficial in this group of patients [27, 32, 33].

The use of vena caval filters instead of anticoagulant treatment in patients with cancer has been evaluated in various trials [34–37]. Although cohort analyses reported apparent beneficial effects of vena caval filters, a large randomized study failed to demonstrate any long-term advantage [34].

Conclusions

Patients with cancer have an enhanced risk of developing venous thromboembolic complications during the course of their disease, especially when they are receiving chemotherapy or when they have recently undergone surgery. Consequently, such patients represent a large subgroup among patients with VTE. The exact incidence of thrombosis in these patients is not well established, however, and the risk contribution according to cancer type and anticancer treatment, as well as a potential beneficial effect of thrombosis prophylaxis, require assessment. Recently, subcutaneous LMWHs have been shown to be at least as safe and efficacious as intravenous UFH in the initial treatment of VTE. The main therapeutic advantages of LMWHs are that monitoring is not required and that only once-daily subcutaneous injections are necessary. Moreover, a meta-analysis of large randomized studies of LMWH versus UFH treatment in cancer and non-cancer patients with VTE has provided preliminary evidence that LMWHs may reduce total mortality in cancer patients. Initiation of treatment with LMWHs in these patients is, therefore, strongly recommended. The usual long-term vitamin K antagonist therapy is more difficult to manage in patients with malignant disease. Compared with non-cancer patients, they appear to be at increased risk for bleeding complications while receiving oral anticoagulant therapy, and frequent laboratory monitoring to maintain a therapeutic range is necessary. Long-term use of LMWHs in therapeutic dosages has not yet been investigated in patients with cancer. Most studies have used prophylactic or subtherapeutic dosages of LMWHs, and have shown similar incidences of VTE recurrence and major bleeding among patients receiving LMWH as among those receiving vitamin K antagonists. Since patients with cancer are already at an increased risk of recurrent VTE, a randomized trial comparing the efficacy and safety of long-term use of LMWH in therapeutic dosages versus conventional-intensity warfarin therapy (INR 2–3) is warranted. Currently, it seems practical to prescribe LMWH in therapeutic dosages to patients with cancer who are difficult to treat with oral anticoagulants.

References

1 Nand S, Fisher SG, Salgia R, Fisher RI: Hemostatic abnormalities in untreated cancer: Incidence and correlation with thrombotic and hemorrhagic complications. J Clin Oncol 1987;5:1998–2003.

2 Pineo GF, Brain MC, Gallus AS, Hirsh J, Hatton MW, Regoeczi E: Tumors, mucus production and hypercoaguability. Ann NY Acad Sci 1974;230:262–270.

3 Ambrus JL, Ambrus CM, Mink IB, Pickren JW: Causes of death in cancer patients. J Med 1975;6:61–64.

4 Rickles FR, Levine M, Edwards RL: Hemostatic alterations in cancer patients. Cancer Metastasis Rev 1992; 11:237–248.

5 Rickles FR, Edwards RL: Activation of blood coagulation in cancer: Trousseau's syndrome revisited. Blood 1983;62:14–31.

6 Nanninga PB, van Teunenbroek A, Veenhof CH, Büller HR, Ten Cate JW: Low prevalence of coagulation and fibrinolytic activation in patients with primary untreated cancer. Thromb Haemost 1990;64: 361–364.

7 Saphner T, Tormey DC, Gray R: Venous and arterial thrombosis in patients who received adjuvant therapy for breast cancer. J Clin Oncol 1991;9:286–294.

8 Fisher B, Costantino J, Redmond C, Poisson R, Bowman D, Couture J, Dimitrov NV, Wolmark N, Wickerham DL, Fisher ER, Margolese R, Robidoux A, Shibata H, Terz J, Paterson AHG, Feldman MI, Farrar W, Evans J, Lickley HL, Ketner M: A randomized clinical trial evaluating tamoxifen in the treatment of patients with node-negative breast cancer who have estrogen-receptor-positive tumors. N Engl J Med 1989; 320:479–484.

9 Clahsen PC, van de Velde CJ, Julien JP, Floiras JL, Mignolet FY: Thromboembolic complications after perioperative chemotherapy in women with early breast cancer: A European Organization for Research and Treatment of Cancer Breast Cancer Cooperative Group study. J Clin Oncol 1994;12:1266–1271.

10 Weiss RB, Tormey DC, Holland JF, Weinberg VE: Venous thrombosis during multimodal treatment of primary breast carcinoma. Cancer Treat Rep 1981;65:677–679.

11 Von Tempelhoff GF, Dietrich M, Hommel G, Heilmann L: Blood coagulation during adjuvant epirubicin/cyclophosphamide chemotherapy in patients with primary operable breast cancer. J Clin Oncol 1996;14: 2560–2568.

12 Rivkin SE, Green S, Metch B, Cruz AB, Adelhoff MD, Jewell WR, Costanzi JJ, Farrar WB, Minton JP, Osborne CK: Adjuvant CMFVP versus tamoxifen versus concurrent CMFVP and tamoxifen for postmenopausal, node-positive, and estrogen receptor-positive breast cancer patients: A Southwest Oncology Group study. J Clin Oncol 1994;12: 2078–2085.

13 Fisher B, Redmond C, Legault-Poisson S, Dimitrov NV, Brown AM, Wickerham DL, Wolmark N, Margolese RG, Bowman D, Glass AG, Kardinal CG, Robidoux A, Jochimsen P, Cronin W, Deutsch M, Fisher ER, Myers DB, Hoehn JL: Postoperative chemotherapy and tamoxifen compared with tamoxifen alone in the treatment of positive-node breast cancer patients aged 50 years and older with tumors responsive to tamoxifen: Results from the National Surgical Adjuvant Breast and Bowel Project B-16. J Clin Oncol 1990;8:1005–1018.

14 Pritchard KI, Paterson AH, Paul NA, Zee B, Fine S, Pater J: Increased thromboembolic complications with concurrent tamoxifen and chemotherapy in a randomized trial of adjuvant therapy for women with breast cancer. National Cancer Institute of Canada Clinical Trials Group Breast Cancer Site Group. J Clin Oncol 1996;14:2731–2737.

15 Goodnough LT, Saito H, Manni A, Jones PK, Pearson OH: Increased incidence of thromboembolism in stage IV breast cancer patients treated with a five-drug chemotherapy regimen. A study of 159 patients. Cancer 1984;54:1264–1268.

16 Levine M, Hirsh J, Gent M, Arnold A, Warr D, Falanga A, Samosh M, Bramwell V, Pritchard KI, Stewart D: Double-blind randomised trial of a very-low-dose warfarin for prevention of thromboembolism in stage IV breast cancer. Lancet 1994; 343:886–889.

17 Brandes AA, Scelzi E, Salmistraro G, Ermani M, Carollo C, Berti F, Zampieri P, Baiocchi C, Fiorentino MV: Incidence of risk of thromboembolism during treatment of high-grade gliomas: A prospective study. Eur J Cancer 1997;33:1592–1596.

18 Cheruku R, Tapazoglou E, Ensley J, Kish JA, Cummings GD, Al-Sarraf M: The incidence and significance of thromboembolic complications in patients with high-grade gliomas. Cancer 1991;68:2621–2624.

19 Levi AD, Wallace MC, Bernstein M, Walters BC: Venous thromboembolism after brain tumor surgery: A retrospective review. Neurosurgery 1991;28:859–863.

20 Von Tempelhoff GF, Dietrich M, Niemann F, Schneider D, Hommel G, Heilmann L: Blood coagulation and thrombosis in patients with ovarian malignancy. Thromb Haemost 1997;77:456–461.

21 Bergqvist D, Burmark US, Flordal PA, Frisell J, Hallbook T, Hedberg D, Horn A, Kelty E, Kvitting P, Lindhagen A: Low molecular weight heparin started before surgery as prophylaxis against deep vein thrombosis: 2,500 versus 5,000 aXa IU in 2,070 patients. Br J Surg 1995; 82:496–501.

22 Hettiarachchi RJK, Prins MH, Lensing AWA, Büller HR: Low molecular weight heparin versus unfractionated heparin in the initial treatment of venous thromboembolism. Curr Opin Pulmon Med 1998; 4:220–225.

23 Hettiarachchi RJK, Smorenburg SM, Ginsberg J, Levine M, Prins MH, Büller HR: Do heparins do more than just treat thrombosis? Thromb Haemost 1999 (in press).

24 Lensing AW, Prins MH, Davidson BL, Hirsh J: Treatment of deep venous thrombosis with low-molecular-weight heparins. A meta-analysis. Arch Intern Med 1995;155:601–607.
25 Hutten BA, Prins MH, Tijssen JGP, Büller HR: The incidence of recurrent thromboembolic and bleeding complications among patients with venous thromboembolism in relation to malignancy and achieved INR (abstract). Thromb Haemost 1997;(suppl):587–588.
26 Bona RD, Hickey AD, Wallace DM: Efficacy and safety of oral anticoagulation in patients with cancer. Thromb Haemost 1997;78:137–140.
27 Prandoni P: Antithrombotic strategies in patients with cancer. Thromb Haemost 1997;78:141–144.
28 Lopaciuk S, Bielska-Falda H, Noszczyk W, Bielawiec M, Witkiewicz M, Filipecki S, Michalak J, Ciesielski L, Mackiewicz Z, Czestochowska E, Zawilska K, Cencora A: Low molecular weight heparin versus acenocoumarol in the secondary prophylaxis of deep vein thrombosis. Thromb Haemost 1999;81:26–31.
29 Pini M, Aiello S, Manotti C, Pattacini C, Quintavalla R, Poli T, Tagliaferri A, Dettori AG: Low molecular weight heparin versus warfarin in the prevention of recurrences after deep vein thrombosis. Thromb Haemost 1994;72:191–197.
30 Das SK, Cohen AT, Edmondson RA, Melissari E, Kakkar VV: Low-molecular-weight heparin versus warfarin for prevention of recurrent venous thromboembolism: A randomized trial. World J Surg 1996; 20:521–526.
31 Monreal M: Alternatives to warfarin in the secondary prevention; in Proceedings of the European Thrombosis Research Organization (ETRO) Working Party on Diagnosis and Treatment of Venous Thromboembolism. Associazione Lotta alla Trombosi. Bologna, 1999.
32 Prins MH, van den Belt AGM, Hutten BA, Bossuyt PMM, Buller HR: Duration of anticoagulant treatment in patients with inherited risk factors; in: Proceedings of the European Thrombosis Research Organization (ETRO) Working Party on Diagnosis and Treatment of Venous Thromboembolism. Associazione Lotta alla Trombosi. Bologna, 1999.
33 Prins MH, Hutten BA, Koopman MWW, Büller HR: Long-term treatment of venous thromboembolic disease. Thromb Haemost 1999, in press.
34 Calligaro KD, Bergen WS, Haut MJ, Savarese RP, DeLaurentis DA: Thromboembolic complications in patients with advanced cancer: Anticoagulation versus Greenfield filter placement. Ann Vasc Surg 1991; 5:186–189.
35 Cohen JR, Tenenbaum N, Citron M: Greenfield filter as primary therapy for deep venous thrombosis and/or pulmonary embolism in patients with cancer. Surgery 1991; 109:12–15.
36 Schwarz RE, Marrero AM, Conlon KC, Burt M: Inferior vena cava filters in cancer patients: Indications and outcome. J Clin Oncol 1996;14: 652–657.
37 Decousus H, Leizorovicz A, Parent F, Page Y, Tardy B, Girard P, Laporte S, Faivre R, Charbonnier B, Barral FG, Huet Y, Simonneau G: A clinical trial of vena caval filters in the prevention of pulmonary embolism in patients with proximal deep-vein thrombosis. N Engl J Med 1998;338:409–415.
38 Levine MN, Gent M, Hirsh J, Arnold A, Goodyear MD, Hryniuk W, De Pauw S: The thrombogenic effect of anticancer drug therapy in women with stage II breast cancer. N Engl J Med 1988;318:404–407.

Workshop 3 Chairmen: J. Conard, J. Ginsberg
Controversies about Anticoagulation during Pregnancy

Hæmostasis

Haemostasis 1999;29(suppl 1):98–104

Management of Pregnancy in Women with Thrombophilia

Jacqueline Conard Marie-Hélène Horellou
Meyer-Michel Samama

Haemostasis-Thrombosis Unit, Hotel-Dieu Hospital, Paris, France

Key Words
Pregnancy · Thrombophilia · Anticoagulation · Heparins

Abstract
Hereditary thrombophilia increases the risk of thrombosis during pregnancy and postpartum. The recommendations resulting from the Fifth American College of Chest Physicians (ACCP) Consensus Conference on Antithrombotic Therapy were published in Chest in late 1998. However, levels of evidence on this subject were low (C2). Furthermore, since publication of this ACCP consensus, new studies have demonstrated the safety of low-molecular-weight heparins (LMWHs) in pregnant women. In addition, it is now clear that all thrombophilias are not associated with the same level of thrombotic risk: factor V Leiden mutation and factor II 20210A variant are associated with a lower risk than antithrombin deficiency. Consequently, the ACCP recommendations have been reconsidered in the light of a more widespread use of LMWH and taking into account the differences in the level of risk of the different thrombophilias. A prophylaxis of thrombosis in pregnant women with thrombophilia is proposed based on published data and our personal experience. Although laboratory monitoring is usually not required during treatments with LMWH, it seems to be needed in pregnant women who receive long-term treatments.

Copyright © 1999 S. Karger AG, Basel

Introduction

Pregnant women have an increased risk of venous thromboembolism (VTE) as compared with non-pregnant women. The risk of thrombosis is further increased by conditions

KARGER

Fax + 41 61 306 12 34
E-Mail karger@karger.ch
www.karger.com

© 1999 S. Karger AG, Basel
0301–0147/99/0297–0098$17.50/0

Accessible online at:
www.karger.com/journals/hae

Dr Jacqueline Conard
Haemostasis-Thrombosis Unit, Hôpital Hôtel-Dieu
Laboratoire Central d'Hématologie
1, Place du Parvis Notre Dame
F–75181 Paris Cedex (France)

such as caesarian section, bed rest during pregnancy, obesity, previous VTE and acquired (lupus anticoagulant) or hereditary coagulation abnormalities (thrombophilia). Consequently, anticoagulant treatment may be indicated during pregnancy. Which anticoagulant is selected for use will depend on its compatibility with pregnancy, the type of thrombophilia and the patient's previous history of thrombosis.

Recommendations of the Fifth American College of Chest Physicians (ACCP) Consensus Conference on Antithrombotic Therapy concerning the prevention and treatment of venous thrombosis in pregnant women were published in Chest in November 1998 [1]. However, new information has since become available which may help in the management of pregnant women with thrombophilia.

Choice of Anticoagulant Treatment

Anticoagulants in common use for the treatment or prevention of venous thrombosis comprise oral anticoagulants (OA), unfractionated heparin (UFH) and low-molecular weight heparins (LMWHs).

Oral Anticoagulants

OA cross the placental barrier and may be responsible for bleeding and teratogenicity in the foetus. The risk of embryopathy (nasal hypoplasia and/or stippled epiphyses) has been shown to be particularly high between 6 and 12 weeks of gestation. In addition, central nervous system abnormalities may occur when OA are given at any time during pregnancy. Finally, cases of serious bleeding have been reported when OA are administered close to delivery.

For these reasons, although OA may still be used during the second trimester in patients with high-risk prosthetic heart valves, they are often completely avoided for the entire duration of the pregnancy.

Unfractionated Heparin

UFH does not cross the placenta and has been considered as the anticoagulant of choice during pregnancy. However, bleeding is still possible and UFH has also some deleterious side effects. It can cause osteoporosis when administered at high doses for long periods; reduction of bone density and fractures have also been observed. In addition, it can induce thrombocytopenia and a decrease in antithrombin. Careful laboratory monitoring is required. UFH can be administered by the intravenous route or by the subcutaneous route: two or three injections are required for the treatment of acute thrombosis, two for prevention.

Low-Molecular-Weight Heparins

LMWHs are increasingly being used for the prevention as well as for the treatment of deep vein thrombosis and pulmonary embolism. Their efficacy and safety have been demonstrated in non-pregnant women. They have the advantage of a longer half-life than UFH, and their high bioavailability allows for once-daily administration for prevention and once- or twice-daily administration for treatment. LMWHs have a more predictable dose response after injection than UFH and therefore can be given without laboratory monitoring. The risk of heparin-induced thrombocytopenia and of osteoporosis are also considered to be lower. Thus, LMWHs are now the treatment of choice for deep vein thrombosis and pulmonary embolism in non-pregnant women, and home treatment is often possible.

LMWHs have been administered to pregnant women as it is thought that LMWH does not cross the placenta, but few studies have been published and most of these have included only small series of patients [2–8]. Just two large series are available [9, 10]. The first one [9] is a review of 486 pregnancies from 21 different studies. Pregnant women received different LMWHs for treatment of an acute episode (5% of cases) or for prophylaxis of thrombosis. In the group of women without comorbid conditions, the frequency of adverse outcome was similar to that seen in the normal population. The second study [10] is a French retrospective multicentre study of 624 pregnancies. The aim of the study was to assess the maternal and foetal safety of enoxaparin, administered for treatment (10%) or for prevention of thrombosis. The conclusions of this study, which included a high proportion of women who were at risk of thrombosis or had previous spontaneous abortions, is that the rate of serious events reasonably related to enoxaparin is low. No unexpected data were found in the mother or in the newborn as compared with the same type of pregnancies in the absence of anticoagulant treatment.

Consequently, if we assume that the efficacy of LMWHs is the same as in nonpregnant women, it is highly suggested that LMWHs are not associated with maternal or foetal adverse events.

Risk of Thrombosis in Thrombophilic Women

The main congenital causes of VTE (thrombophilia) are: deficiency in antithrombin (AT; previously named AT III), protein C (PC) or protein S (PS), activated protein C (APC) resistance associated with factor V Leiden mutation, and prothrombin 20210A variant [11, 12]. Hyperhomocysteinaemia, homozygosity for methylene tetrahydrofolate reductase and increased levels of factor VIII may also be considered as risk factors.

Thrombophilias are all associated with an increased risk of VTE but their frequency and severity differ. Indeed, factor V Leiden mutation is the most common abnormality in Caucasian subjects, present in 20% of unselected patients with venous thrombosis and in about 5% of the general population; AT deficiency is much less frequent (about 1% of patients) [11].

Probands with thrombophilia are usually studied because they have had thrombotic episodes. The study of their relatives who are also carriers of thrombophilia is more appropriate for the elevation of the real risk of thrombosis associated thrombophilia. Recently, a retrospective cohort family study has focused on 513 relatives from 233 thrombophilic families in which the proband had at least one VTE episode [13]. The aim of the study was to assess the risk of VTE in individuals with AT, PC or PS deficiency, or APC resistance. The overall incidence of VTE (per 100 patient-years) in the relatives was 0.52; however, the incidence was higher in those with AT deficiency (1.07) than in those with PC (0.54) or PS (0.50) deficiency, whereas persons with APC resistance had the lowest incidence (0.30). Women had the peak incidence at a younger age than men (21–40 years versus 41–60 years). The first episode was frequently associated with oral contraceptives (11%) or puerperium (21%). The risk related to the prothrombin 20210A variant has not yet been clearly determined but it seems close to the risk of factor V Leiden.

In the absence of anticoagulant prophylaxis, the risk of deep vein thrombosis or pulmonary embolism (exclusion of superficial vein thrombosis) related to pregnancy and postpartum has been shown to be 24–28% in women with AT, PC or PS deficiency (table 1). AT-deficient women have a high risk during pregnancy (14–40%) and postpartum (11–26%), while PS-deficient women have a very

Table 1. Risk of deep vein thrombosis and pulmonary embolism related to pregnancy in women with AT, PC or PS deficiency

	Women	Pregnancies	VTE, %
Conard et al., 1990 [14]	77	155	37 (24)
Pabinger and Schneider, 1996 [15]	71	176	49 (28)
Friederich et al., 1996[1] [16]	60	169	7 (4)
Non-carriers	69	198	1 (0.5)

1 Relatives only, no previous VTE.

Table 2. Risk of deep vein thrombosis and pulmonary embolism related to pregnancy in women with AT, PC or PS deficiency

	AT, %	PC, %	PS, %
VTE during pregnancy			
Conard et al., 1990 [14]	14	4	0
Pabinger and Schneider, 1996 [15]	40	10	6
Friederich et al., 1996 [16]	3	2	0
VTE postpartum			
Conard et al., 1990 [14]	26	17	13
Pabinger and Scheider, 1996 [15]	11	5	22
Friederich et al., 1996 [16]	0	0	7

low risk during pregnancy (0–6%) but are at a greatly increased risk in the postpartum period (13–22%) [14, 15] (table 2). In these two studies [14, 15], women were either the probands or the relatives and were included irrespective of whether they had had a previous thrombosis before pregnancy or not. In another study [16], which included only relatives without a history of thrombosis, the incidence was much lower but still increased as compared with the normal population. The risk reported is lower in women with factor V Leiden mutation than in AT-, PC- or PS-deficient carriers (RR 4.2, 95% CI 0.5–148 versus RR 8.2, 95% CI 1.2–184) [17]. The incidence of VTE was similar in two studies of families with factor V Leiden mutation [17, 18].

There is evidence that VTE is more common in the postpartum period than during pregnancy and is more common in the last trimester of pregnancy than in the first or second trimester. In some studies, women who had VTE during the first trimester may not have been excluded for calculation of the risk during the second or third trimester, leading to an underestimation of the risk in the last trimester. The same may be responsible for the lower risk in postpartum found in some studies.

In summary, pregnant women with thrombophilia are at higher risk of deep vein thrombosis and pulmonary embolism than pregnant women in the general population, and the risk is likely to be higher in the postpartum period than during pregnancy.

Prevention of Thromboembolism in Pregnant Women with Thrombophilia

The 1998 ACCP recommendations have been published in Chest [1]. However, all those concerning women with previous VTE and/or thrombophilia were grade C2 (i.e. weak); furthermore, new information has become available lately. Consequently, we will make some comments taking into account the new information and our personal experience.

General Recommendations

In all pregnant women with thrombophilia, with or without a history of VTE, a clinical surveillance is recommended. The advice of an angiologist is useful to evaluate the venous status, determine whether a compression ultrasound or the use of elastic stockings are required.

There is also a consensus to recommend heparin or warfarin for 4 to 6 weeks postpartum in all pregnant women at risk of thrombosis.

Women with a History of VTE Prior to the Current Pregnancy

Chest recommendations are prophylaxis using adjusted-dose subcutaneous heparin throughout pregnancy. The dose is adjusted to produce a heparin level (anti-factor Xa activity) of 0.1 to 0.2 IU/ml. A dose of 5,000 IU every 12 h is considered as probably insufficient. The use of LMWH is suggested but no information is given concerning the dose to be administered and the requirement for laboratory monitoring. In women with a previous VTE in association with a transient risk factor, the authors suggest a clinical surveillance may be sufficient.

We feel that a similar prophylactic regimen for all pregnant women with a previous history of VTE, with or without thrombophilia, is not appropriate. Women with AT deficiency are at high risk and probably require a more active prophylaxis: we usually recommend twice-daily administration of LMWH at a dose level sufficient to obtain an anti-Xa activity of 0.3 to 0.4 IU/ml at 3 to 4 h after injection. In contrast, the risk is probably lower in women with factor V Leiden mutation and it may be questioned whether clinical surveillance and elastic stockings throughout pregnancy and LMWH once a day during the third trimester only might be sufficient in such patients. These ideas have not been validated in clinical trials but we should remember that there is no solid evidence for the recommendations of *Chest* either.

Pregnancy in Women on Long-Term Anticoagulant Therapy

Because of the high risk of warfarin embryopathy between 6 and 12 weeks of gestation, and assuming there is no risk before the 6th week, women are counselled to perform a pregnancy test as soon as possible. If the test is positive, heparin is substituted for oral anticoagulants. Replacement of oral anticoagulants with heparin before conception had been proposed, but, as this would prolong the duration of exposure to heparin and, consequently, increase the risk of osteoporosis, this option has since been abandoned.

Thrombophilic Women Without a Personal History of VTE

Chest recommendations are clinical surveillance or low-dose heparin (either 5,000 IU every 12 h subcutaneously or adjusted to produce a heparin level of 0.1 to 0.2 IU/ml) throughout pregnancy.

We feel that clinical surveillance is probably sufficient in women with protein S deficiency and in heterozygous carriers of factor V Leiden mutation or prothrombin 20210A variant but does not seem appropriate for women with AT deficiency. In the latter, at least low doses of LMWH (4,000–5,000 IU) once a day are probably required throughout pregnancy, in order to achieve anti-factor Xa activity levels of 0.20–0.40 IU/ml at 3–4 h after the injection. These doses have been proposed in women who have no known thrombophilia but have had a previous thrombosis [7].

Conclusion

The management of thrombophilic women during pregnancy is not yet well determined. Recommendations of the ACCP Consensus Conference are generally appropriate although they have not individualized the thrombophilias and concern mainly UFH. It is now clear that all thrombophilias are not the same and differ in severity. LMWHs are widely used in non-pregnant women and seem to be safe during pregnancy.

Because of the absence of a clear consensus, the management of thrombophilic pregnant women requires the help of different medical specialties (gynaecology, haematology, internal medicine). The anticoagulant used must be adapted to pregnancy, the intensity and duration of the treatment and to the type of thrombophilia.

References

1 Ginsberg JS, Hirsh J: Use of antithrombotic agents during pregnancy. Chest 1998;114:S524–S530.
2 Gillis S, Shushan A, Eldor A: Use of low molecular weight heparin for prophylaxis and treatment of thromboembolism in pregnancy. Int J Gynaecol Obstet 1992;39:297–301.
3 Hellgren M, Bremme K, Blomback M, Siegbahn A: Thromboprophylaxis with Fragmin during pregnancy. Acta Obstet Gynecol Scand 1996; 75(suppl 162):86.
4 Hunt BJ, Doughty HA, Majumdar G, Copplestone A, Kerslake S, Buchanan N: Thromboprophylaxis with low molecular weight heparin (Fragmin) in high risk pregnancies. Thomb Haemost 1997;77:39–43.
5 Nelson-Piercy C, Letsky EA, de Swiet M: Low molecular weight heparin for obstetric thromboprophylaxis: Experience of sixty-nine pregnancies in sixty-one women at high risk. Am J Obstet Gynecol 1997; 176:1062–1068.
6 Horellou MH, Conard J, Achkar A, Miserey G, Hadjez JM, Elalamy I, Samama M: Treatment of thrombosis with low molecular weight heparins during 15 pregnancies in 14 women. Thromb Haemost 1997, suppl, p 733.
7 Blombäck M, Bremme K, Hellgren M, Siegbahn A, Lindberg H: Thromboprophylaxis with low molecular mass heparin, 'Fragmin' (dalteparin), during pregnancy – a longitudinal safety study. Blood Coagul Fibrinol 1998;9:1–9.
8 Brennand JE, Walker ID, Greer IA: Anti-activated factor X profiles in pregnant women receiving antenatal prophylaxis with enoxaparin. Acta Haematol 1999;101:53–55.
9 Sanson BJ, Lensing AWA, Prins MH, Ginsberg JS, Barkagan ZS, Lavenne-Pardonge E, Brenner B, Dulitzky M, Nielsen JD, Boda Z, Turi S, MacGillavry MR, Hamulyak K, Theunissen IM, Hun BJ, Büller HR: Safety of low-molecular-weight heparin in pregnancy: A systematic review. Thromb Haemost 1999;81:668–672.
10 Borel-Derlon A, Borg JY, Boudignat O, Cohen C, Conard J, Francoual C, Lepercq J, Priollet P, Schved JF, Steinberg G, Tournaire M, Yvelin N: Assessment of a low molecular weight heparin (enoxaparin) safety during pregnancy; a retrospective study of 624 pregnancies. Thromb Haemost 1999;suppl:491.
11 Lane DA, Mannucci PM, Bauer KA, Bertina RM, Bochkov NP, Boulyjenkov V, Chandy M, Dahlback B, Ginter EK, Miletich JP, Rosendaal FR, Seligsohn U: Inherited thrombophilia: Part 1. Thromb Haemost 1996;76:651–662.
12 Lane DA, Mannucci PM, Bauer KA, Bertina RM, Bochkov NP, Boulyjenkov V, Chandy M, Dahlback B, Ginter EK, Miletich JP, Rosendaal FR, Seligsohn U: Inherited thrombophilia: Part 2. Thromb Haemost 1996;76:824–834.

13 Bucciarelli P, Rosendaal FR, Tripodi A, Mannucci M, De Stefano V, Palareti G, Finazzi G, Baudo F, Quintavilla R, on behalf of the GIRTE (Italian Research Group on Inherited Thrombophilia): Risk of venous thromboembolism and clinical manifestations in carriers of antithrombin, protein C, protein S deficiency, or activated protein C resistance: A multicentre collaborative family study. Arterioscler Thromb Vasc Biol 1999;19:1026–1033.
14 Conard J, Horellou MH, Van Dreden P, Lecompte T, Samama M: Thrombosis and pregnancy in congenital deficiencies in AT III, protein C or protein S: Study of 78 women. Thromb Haemost 1990;63: 319–320.
15 Pabinger I, Schneider B: Thrombotic risk in hereditary antithrombin III, protein C and protein S deficiency. Arterioscl Thromb Vasc Biol 1996;16:742–748.
16 Friederich PW, Sanson BJ, Simioni P, Zanardi S, Huisman MV, Kindt I, Prandoni P, Büller HR, Girolami A, Prins MH: Frequency of pregnancy related venous thromboembolism in anticoagulant factor deficient women: Implications for prophylaxis. Ann Intern Med 1996;125: 955–960.
17 Simioni P, Sanson BJ, Prandoni P, Tormene D, Friederich PW, Girolami B, Gavasso S, Huisman MV, Büller HR, ten Cate JW, Girolami A, Prins MH: Incidence of venous thromboembolism in families with inherited thrombophilia. Thromb Haemost 1998;81:198–202.
18 Middeldorp S, Henkens CMA, Koopman MMW, Van Pampus ECM, Hamulyak K, Van der Meer J, Prins MH, Büller HR: The incidence of venous thromboembolism in family members of patients with factor V Leiden mutation and venous thrombosis. Ann Intern Med 1998;128:15–20.

Workshop 3 Chairmen: J. Conard, J. Ginsberg
Controversies about Anticoagulation during Pregnancy

Haemostasis

Haemostasis 1999;29(suppl 1):105–106

What Is the Optimal Management of Pregnant Women with Valvular Heart Disease in Pregnancy?

Wee Shian Chan

Department of Internal Medicine (Obstetrical Medicine), Women's College Hospital, Toronto, Ont., Canada

Key Words
Anticoagulation · Mechanical heart valve · Thrombosis · Pregnancy

Abstract
Women with mechanical heart valves require anticoagulation during pregnancy. Continued anticoagulation with coumadin throughout the first trimester can result in foetopathic effects in 6.4% (95% CI, 4.6–8.9%) of cases. Replacement of warfarin with heparin between 6 and 12 weeks' gestation eliminates this risk. Although warfarin does cross the placenta, adverse central nervous system effects associated with its use are very few. Warfarin is effective in preventing maternal thromboembolic complications, while the effectiveness of heparin in preventing valve thrombosis is unproven. The optimal management (grade C2 recommendation) of women with mechanical heart valves may involve the use of warfarin throughout pregnancy except for two time periods – between 6 and 12 weeks' gestation and after 36 weeks of gestation. During these times, adjusted-dose unfractionated heparin should be used to rigorously maintain a therapeutic mid-interval activated partial thromboplastin time of 2.0 to 2.5 times the control. The additional use of low-dose aspirin should be considered, particularly in women with high-risk valves, women with previous transient ischaemic attacks and/or strokes, and women with atrial fibrillation.

Copyright © 1999 S. Karger AG, Basel

The management of women with prosthetic heart valves in pregnancy poses a particular challenge for clinicians and their patients because of the lack of controlled studies. While the management of pregnant women with biological valve replacements is relatively clear, the management of pregnant women with mechanical heart valves has been controversial [1, 2].

The use of oral anticoagulants (OA) such as warfarin results in the characteristic warfarin embryopathy during first-trimester exposure; further exposure of the foetus to the drug beyond the first trimester is reported to result in other adverse events involving the central

KARGER

Fax + 41 61 306 12 34
E-Mail karger@karger.ch
www.karger.com

© 1999 S. Karger AG, Basel
0301–0147/99/0297–0105$17.50/0

Accessible online at:
www.karger.com/journals/hae

Dr. Wee Shian Chan
Department of Internal Medicine, Obstetrical Medicine
Women's College Hospital, Burton Hall
60 Grosvenor Street, Suite 424
Toronto, Ont. M5S 1B6 (Canada)

nervous system [3]. The effectiveness of heparin in preventing valve thrombosis has been brought into question from multiple case reports of therapy failure and adverse maternal outcomes [4–6].

A systematic review of the literature [7] has provided estimates of maternal and foetal risks associated with three commonly used approaches: (1) OA throughout pregnancy, (2) replacing OA with heparin from 6–12 weeks, and (3) heparin use throughout pregnancy.

Exposure of the foetus to OA in the first trimester was associated with congenital anomalies in 6.4% (95% CI, 4.6–8.9%) of live births [7]. The most common manifestation, in 70% of cases, was warfarin embryopathy, consisting of nasal hypoplasia and epiphysis stippling. The substitution of heparin at or prior to 6 weeks and continued until 12 weeks eliminated this risk. The overall risk of foetal wastage (spontaneous loss, stillbirths and neonatal deaths) was similar in women treated with OA throughout as compared with women treated with heparin in the first trimester. Maternal mortality in women with mechanical heart valves was significant compared with overall maternal mortality, at 2.9% (95% CI, 1.9–4.3%) [7]. The most common cause (68%) of maternal mortality was thrombosis of the mechanical valves. Major bleeding associated with anticoagulation occurred in 2.5% (95% CI, 1.7–3.5%) of all pregnancies, mostly occurring at the time of delivery [7].

The regimen associated with the lowest risk of valve thrombosis (3.9%; 95% CI, 2.9–5.9%) was the use of OA throughout. Using heparin only between 6 and 12 weeks' gestation was associated with an increased risk of valve thrombosis (9.2%; 95% CI 5.9–13.9%).

In conclusion, our view of the literature [7] would suggest the following: (1) the use of OA throughout pregnancy, although providing optimal thromboembolic prophylaxis of women with mechanical heart valves in pregnancy; however, this increases the risk of foetal embryopathy. (2) Replacing OA with heparin between 6 and 12 weeks will reduce the risk of foetopathic effects but subjects the woman to an increased risk of thromboembolic complications. (3) The use of low-dose subcutaneous heparin is inadequate; the use of adjusted-dose heparin warrants aggressive monitoring and appropriate dose adjustment. Large prospective trials to determine the best regimen, the role of low-molecular-weight heparin and the benefit of adding an antiplatelet agent [8] in these women with mechanical valves are urgently needed.

References

1 Sbarouni E, Oakley CM: Outcome of pregnancy in women with valve prostheses. Br Heart J 1994;71:196–201.
2 Ginsberg JS, Barron WM: Pregnancy and prosthetic heart valves. Lancet 1994;344:1170–1172.
3 Hall JG, Pauli RM, Wilson KM: Maternal and fetal sequelae of anticoagulation during pregnancy. Am J Med 1980;68:122–140.
4 Golby AJ, Bush EC, DeRook FA, Albers GW: Failure of high dose heparin to prevent recurrent cardioembolic strokes in a pregnant patient with a mechanical heart valve. Neurology 1992;42:2204–2206.
5 Watson WJ, Freeman J, O'Brien C, Benson M: Embolic stroke in a pregnant patient with a mechanical heart valve on optimal heparin therapy. Am J Perinatol 1996;36:371–372.
6 Hurwitz A, Milwidsky A, Medina A, Yagel S: Failure of continuous intravenous heparinization to prevent stroke in a pregnant woman with a prosthetic valve and atrial fibrillation. J Reprod Med 1985;30:618–620.
7 Chan WS, Anand S, Ginsberg JS: Anticoagulation of pregnant women with mechanical heart valves: A systematic review of the literature. Arch Intern Med (in press).
8 Turpie AG, Gent M, Laupacis A, Latour Y, Gunstensen J, Basile F, Klimek M, Hirsh J: A comparison of aspirin and placebo in patients treated with warfarin after heart-valve replacement. N Engl J Med 1993;329:524–529.

Workshop 3 Chairmen: J. Conard, J. Ginsberg
Controversies about Anticoagulation during Pregnancy

Hæmostasis

Haemostasis 1999;29(suppl 1):107–111

Optimal Management of Pregnant Women with Acute Venous Thromboembolism

Shannon M. Bates

Department of Medicine, McMaster University and Hamilton Civic Hospitals Research Center, Hamilton, Ont., Canada

Key Words
Pregnancy · Thrombosis · Treatment · Heparin · Warfarin · Low-molecular-weight heparin

Abstract
Venous thromboembolism (VTE) is an important cause of obstetric morbidity and mortality. Its management during pregnancy is problematic because anticoagulants, the cornerstone of initial therapy for VTE, may have significant foetal as well as maternal side effects. Unfractionated heparin has been the anticoagulant of choice in pregnancy; however, there is growing clinical experience with low-molecular-weight heparin (LMWH) in this patient population. A recently published systematic review of the literature suggests that the use of LMWH during pregnancy is not associated with adverse foetal/infant outcomes. Moreover, its long-term use appears to be safe for the mother, as symptomatic osteoporosis, bleeding and heparin-induced thrombocytopenia occurred only infrequently. There are limited data regarding the efficacy of anticoagulant therapy in the treatment of VTE during pregnancy, and treatment recommendations have largely been extrapolated from data in non-pregnant patients and case series of pregnant patients. This paper will briefly review the challenges and areas of controversy associated with the use of anticoagulants in the treatment of pregnancy-associated VTE.

Copyright © 1999 S. Karger AG, Basel

Although venous thromboembolism (VTE) is an uncommon complication of pregnancy, it is the leading cause of maternal morbidity and mortality [1, 2]. Evidence for the efficacy

KARGER

Fax + 41 61 306 12 34
E-Mail karger@karger.ch
www.karger.com

© 1999 S. Karger AG, Basel
0301–0147/99/0297–0107$17.50/0

Accessible online at:
www.karger.com/journals/hae

Dr. S.M. Bates
Department of Medicine
McMaster University and Hamilton Civic Hospitals Research Center
711 Concession Street
Hamilton, Ont. L8V 1C3 (Canada)

of anticoagulant therapy in the treatment of VTE comes from a randomized trial involving non-pregnant patients with clinically suspected pulmonary embolism [3] and a literature review of maternal mortality secondary to pulmonary embolism [4]. The use of anticoagulants during pregnancy remains problematic because they may produce complications in both the foetus and the mother.

Warfarin

Warfarin, the most commonly used oral anticoagulant, crosses the placenta [5, 6] and has been associated with warfarin embryopathy and abnormalities of the central nervous system [7–11]. Neonatal haemorrhage is a possibility if coumarin derivatives are administered to the mother near term [6, 12]. Although warfarin embryopathy has been reported to occur in up to 30% of infants exposed to warfarin between 6 and 12 weeks of gestation [13], other workers have suggested that the incidence more likely approximates 5% [11, 14]. Central nervous system abnormalities have been reported in 3% of pregnancies associated with oral anticoagulant therapy [11, 14].

Unfractionated Heparin (UFH)

UFH does not cross the placenta [15] and would not be expected to produce foetal complications. Two publications [14, 16] confirm that UFH is relatively safe for the foetus. In a cohort study of 100 consecutive pregnancies associated with UFH therapy [16], the rate of bleeding was consistent with that reported during the treatment of VTE in non-pregnant patients [17, 18]. A prolonged anticoagulant effect at the time of delivery [19], heparin-induced thrombocytopenia [20, 21], the need for laboratory monitoring with regular dose adjustments [22], and heparin-associated osteoporosis [23–31] are drawbacks associated with the use of UFH.

Low-Molecular-Weight Heparin (LMWH)

In non-pregnant patients with VTE, LMWHs and UFH have equivalent safety and efficacy [32]. The increased half-life and improved bioavailability of LMWH [33, 34] permit once-daily weight-adjusted subcutaneous dosing. A predictable anticoagulant response obviates the need for routine monitoring [35]. LMWHs are also associated with a lower incidence of heparin-induced thrombocytopenia [36]. On the basis of the limited information available, the risk of osteoporosis also appears to be less with LMWH [37–39]. LMWH does not cross the placental barrier [38, 40].

The evaluation of LMWHs in pregnancy has been limited to small case series. A recent systematic review evaluated a total of 486 pregnancies from 21 different studies [41] and concluded that the observed rate of adverse outcomes in women without comorbid conditions was similar to that observed when a comparable evaluation was performed in pregnant women receiving UFH [14]. This suggests that the use of LMWH is not associated with adverse foetal/infant outcomes. Although symptomatic osteoporosis, bleeding and heparin-induced thrombocytopenia occurred infrequently, only 5% of women were treated with therapeutic doses of LMWH and it is possible that higher doses might be associated with an increased risk of these complications. Moreover, only three of the studies systematically evaluated bone density. VTE occurred in 0.6% of all pregnancies, suggesting that LMWH provides effective prophylaxis, but not all women were at increased risk of this complication. Definite conclusions about the effectiveness of LMWH in the treatment of VTE cannot be drawn from this study.

Treatment Recommendations

There are limited data regarding the efficacy of anticoagulant therapy in the treatment of VTE during pregnancy. Recommendations have been extrapolated from data in non-pregnant patients and case series of pregnant women (C2 guidelines from the American College of Chest Physicians) [42]. Pregnant patients with objectively documented VTE should be treated with either UFH or LMWH.

Initial therapy has traditionally consisted of a bolus of intravenous UFH followed by a continuous infusion adjusted to maintain a therapeutic activated partial thromboplastin time (APTT). On the basis of the results from two studies [16, 43], intravenous heparin is discontinued and therapy with twice-daily subcutaneous UFH, in doses sufficient to achieve a therapeutic mid-interval APTT, is commenced after 5–10 days. The APTT should be checked every few weeks because UFH requirements might vary as the pregnancy progresses. Apparent heparin resistance during pregnancy is not uncommon and monitoring of heparin levels by anti-factor Xa assay has been suggested [44]. Despite validation of this approach in non-pregnant patients [45], similar data are lacking in the pregnant population. Although there is growing clinical experience with LMWH in pregnancy, good information on appropriate dosage regimens and the need for dose adjustment or laboratory monitoring is lacking. Anticoagulant therapy should be continued throughout pregnancy and for 4–6 weeks after delivery. If the episode of VTE occurs late in the pregnancy, at least 3 months of anticoagulant therapy should be administered. Warfarin, which is safe for breast-feeding infants [46, 47], can be substituted following delivery.

A prolonged anticoagulant effect at the time of delivery may increase the risk of bleeding or haematoma formation with epidural analgesia [19]. Planned delivery is often advocated, with discontinuation of subcutaneous UFH or LMWH 24 h prior to elective induction. Women at high risk of recurrent thromboembolism can be converted to an infusion of UFH that is discontinued 4–6 h prior to delivery. Women with spontaneous onset of labour should discontinue injections immediately. The APTT must be checked to ensure it has normalized with discontinuation of UFH. If necessary, rapid reversal of heparinization in patients receiving UFH can be accomplished with protamine sulphate. The optimal approach in women who enter spontaneous labour while receiving therapeutic doses of LMWH remains controversial and depends upon the proximity of the last dose to the expected time of delivery, and, if available, the anti-factor Xa level. If a significant anticoagulant effect is expected or documented at the time of delivery, epidural analgesia should be avoided and protamine sulphate should be used judiciously. After delivery, therapeutic doses of UFH or LMWH should be reintroduced with adequate haemostasis. Warfarin can be started immediately and heparin discontinued once the international normalized ratio has been in the therapeutic range for two consecutive days.

At present, it is our practice to use weight-adjusted doses that are increased as the woman's weight increases. The need for measurement of anti-factor Xa concentrations remains controversial.

References

1 Franks AI, Atrash HK, Lawson HW, Colberg KS: Obstetrical pulmonary embolism mortality, United States 1970–1985. Am J Public Health 1990;80:720–722.

2 Rochat RW, Koonin LM, Atrash HK, Jewett JF: Maternal mortality in the United States: Report from the Maternal Mortality Collaborative. Obstet Gynecol 1988;72:91–97.

3 Barritt DW, Jordan SC: Anticoagulant drugs in the treatment of pulmonary embolism: A controlled trial. Lancet 1960;i:1309–1312.

4 Villasanta U: Thromboembolic disease in pregnancy. Am J Obstet Gynecol 1965;93:142–160.

5 Quick AJ: Experimentally induced changes in the prothrombin level of the blood. III. Prothrombin concentration of newborn pups of a mother given dicoumarol before parturition. J Biol Chem 1946;164:371–376.

6 Kraus AP, Perlow A, Singer K: Danger of dicoumarol treatment in pregnancy. J Am Med Assoc 1949;139: 758–782.

7 DiSaia PJ: Pregnancy and delivery of a patient with a Starr-Edwards mitral valve prosthesis: Report of a case. Obstet Gynecol 1966;28:469–472.

8 Kerber IJ, Warr OS, Richardson C: Pregnancy in a patient with a prosthetic mitral valve. J Am Med Assoc 1968;203:223–225.

9 Becker HM, Genieser NB, Finegold M, Miranda D, Spackman T: Chrondroplasia punctata: Is maternal warfarin a factor? Am J Dis Child 1975:129:356–359.

10 Shaul WL, Hall JG: Multiple congenital anomalies associated with oral anticoagulants. Am J Obstet Gynecol 1977;27:191–198.

11 Hall JAG, Paul RM, Wilson KM: Maternal and fetal sequelae of anticoagulation during pregnancy. Am J Med 1980;68:122–140.

12 Hirsh J, Cade JF, Gallus AS: Fetal effects of Coumadin administered during pregnancy. Blood 1970;36: 623–627.

13 Iturbe-Alessio I, del Carment Fonseca M, Mutchinik O, Santos MA, Zajarias A, Salazar E: Risks of anticoagulant therapy in pregnant women with artificial heart valves. N Engl J Med 1986;315:1390–1393.

14 Ginsberg JS, Hirsh J, Turner C, Levine MN, Burrows R: Risks to the fetus of anticoagulant therapy during pregnancy. Thromb Haemost 1989;61:197–203.

15 Flessa HC, Kapstrom AB, Glueck MJ, Will JJ: Placental transport of heparin. Am J Obstet Gynecol 1965; 93:570–573.

16 Ginsberg J, Kowalchuk G, Hirsh J, Brill-Edwards P, Burrows R: Heparin therapy during pregnancy: Risks to the fetus and mother. Arch Intern Med 1989:149:2233–2236.

17 Hull R, Delmore T, Carter C, Hirsh J, Genton E, Gent M, Turpie G, McLaughlin D: Adjusted subcutaneous heparin versus warfarin sodium in the long-term treatment of venous thrombosis. N Engl J Med 1982:306;189–194.

18 Hull R, Hirsh J, Jay R, Carter C, Gent M, Turpie AGG, McLoughlin D, Dodd P, Thomas M, Raskob G, Ockleford P: Different intensities of oral anticoagulant therapy in the treatment of proximal vein thrombosis. N Engl J Med 1982;307: 1676–1681.

19 Anderson DR, Ginsberg JS, Burrows R, Brill-Edwards P: Subcutaneous heparin therapy during pregnancy: A need for concern at the time of delivery. Thromb Haemost 1991;65:248–250.

20 Kapsch D, Silver D: Heparin-induced thrombocytopenia with thrombosis and hemorrhage. Arch Surg 1981;116:1423–1427.

21 Aster RH: Heparin-induced thrombocytopenia and thrombosis. N Engl J Med 1995;332:1374–1376.

22 Hirsh J, Fuster V: Guide to anticoagulant therapy. Part 1: Heparin. Circulation 1994;89:1449–1468.

23 Griffith GC, Nichol G, Asher JD, Hanagan B: Heparin osteoporosis. J Am Med Assoc 1965;193:191–194.

24 Dahlman TC, Sjoberg HE, Ringertz H: Bone mineral density during long-term prophylaxis with heparin in pregnancy. Am J Obstet Gynecol 1994;160:1315–1320.

25 Dahlman TC, Hellgren MS, Blomback M: Thrombosis prophylaxis in pregnancy with use of subcutaneous heparin adjusted by monitoring heparin concentration in plasma. Am J Obstet Gynecol 1989;161: 420–425.

26 Dahlman TC: Osteoporotic fractures and the recurrence of thromboembolism during pregnancy and the puerperium in 184 women undergoing thromboprophylaxis with heparin. Am J Obstet Gynecol 1993; 168:1265–1270.

27 Howell R, Fidler J, Letsky E, De Swiet M: The risks of antenatal subcutaneous heparin prophylaxis: a controlled trial. Br J Obstet Gynaecol 1983;30:1124–1128.

28 Ginsberg JS, Kowalchuk G, Hirsh J, Brill-Edwards P, Burrows R, Coates G, Webber C: Heparin effect on bone density. Thromb Haemost 1990;64:286–289.

29 Dalham T, Lindall N, Hellgren M: Osteopenia in pregnancy during long-term heparin treatment: A radiological study postpartum. Br J Obstet Gynaecol 1990;97:221–228.

30 Barbour LA, Kick SD, Steiner JF, LoVerde ME, Heddleston LN, Lear JL: A prospective study of heparin-induced osteoporosis using bone densitometry. Am J Obstet Gynecol 1994;170:862–869.

31 Douketis JD, Ginsberg JS, Burows RD, Duku EK, Webber CE, Brill-Edwards P: The effect of long-term heparin therapy on bone density: A prospective matched cohort study. Thromb Haemost 1996;75:254–257.

32 Gould MK, Dembitzer AD, Doyle RL, Hastie TJ, Garber AM: Low-molecular-weight heparins compared with unfractionated heparin for treatment of acute deep venous thrombosis: A meta-analysis of randomized, controlled trials. Ann Intern Med 1999;130:800–809.

33 Bara L, Billaud E, Gramond G, Kher A, Samama M: Comparative pharmacokinetics of a low-molecular-weight heparin (PK 10169) and unfractionated heparin after intravenous and subcutaneous administration. Thromb Res 1985;39:631–636.
34 Bara L, Samama M: Pharmacokinetics of low molecular weight heparins. Acta Chir Scand Suppl 1988; 543:65–72.
35 Weitz J: Low-molecular-weight heparins. N Engl J Med 1997;337:688–698.
36 Warkentin TE, Levine MN, Hirsh J, Horsewood P, Roberts RS, Gent M, Kelton JG: Heparin-induced thrombocytopenia in patients treated with low-molecular-weight heparin or unfractionated heparin. N Engl J Med 1995;332:1330–1335.
37 Monreal M, Lafoz E, Live A, de Rio L, Vedia C: Comparison of subcutaneous unfractionated heparin with a low molecular weight heparin (Fragmin) in patients with venous thromboembolism and contraindications for coumarin. Thromb Haemost 1994;71:7–11.
38 Melissari E, Parker CJ, Wilson NV, Monte G, Kanthou C, Pemberton KD, Nicolaides KH, Barrett JJ, Kakkar VV: Use of low molecular weight heparin in pregnancy. Thromb Haemost 1992;68:652–656.
39 Sefras J, Farquahrson RG: Bone density studies in pregnant women receiving heparin. Eur J Obstet Gynecol Reprod Biol 1996;65:171–174.
40 Forestier F, Daffos F, Rainaut M, Toulemonde F: Low-molecular-weight-heparin (CY 216) does not cross the placenta during the third trimester of pregnancy. Thromb Haemost 1987;57:234.
41 Sanson B, Lensing AWA, Prins MH, Ginsberg JS, Barkagan ZS, Lavenne-Pardonge E, Brenner B, Dulitzky M, Nielsen JD, Boda Z, Turi S, MacGillavry MR, Hamulyak K, Theunissen IM, Hunt BJ, Buller HR: The use of low-molecular-weight heparin in pregnancy: A systematic review. Thromb Haemost 1999;81:668–672.
42 Ginsberg JS, Hirsh J: Use of antithrombotic agents during pregnancy. Chest 1998;114(suppl):524–530.
43 Hull R, Delmore T, Genton E, Hirsh J, Gent M, Sackett D, McLoughlin D, Armstrong P: Warfarin sodium versus low-dose heparin in the long-term treatment of venous thrombosis. N Engl J Med 1979;301:855–858.
44 Lowe GDO: Treatment of venous thromboembolism; in Greer IA (ed): Baillière's Clinical Obstetrics and Gynaecology – Thromboembolic Disease in Obstetrics and Gynaecology. London, Baillière Tindall, 1997, pp 511–521.
45 Levine MN, Hirsh J, Gent M, Turpie AG, Cruikshank M, Weitz J, Anderson D, Johnson M: A randomized trial comparing activated thromboplastin time with heparin assay in patients with acute venous thromboembolism requiring large daily doses of heparin. Arch Intern Med 1994;154:49–56.
46 Orme ML, Lewis M, DeSwiet M, Serlin MJ, Sibeon R, Baty JD, Breckenridge AM: May mothers given warfarin breast-feed their infants? Br Med J 1977;1:1564–1565.
47 McKenna R, Cole ER, Vasan U: Is warfarin sodium contraindicated in the lactating mother? J Pediatr 1983;103:325–327.

Workshop 3 Chairmen: J. Conard, J. Ginsberg
Controversies about Anticoagulation during Pregnancy

Hæmostasis

Haematosis 1999;29(suppl 1):112–120

Is there a Role for Antithrombotic Therapy in the Prevention of Pregnancy Loss?

Bertrand Wechsler Lê Thi Huong Du Jean Charles Piette

Department of Internal Medicine, Groupe Hospitalier Pitié-Salpêtrière, Paris, France

Key Words
Pregnancy loss · Antiphospholipid syndrome · Heparin · Aspirin · Steroids · Infertility

Abstract
The antiphospholipid syndrome (APS) is now emerging as an important cause of recurrent pregnancy loss. A variety of treatments, including steroids, aspirin, heparin and immunoglobulin, alone or in combination, have been assessed in experimental studies and in clinical trials. Steroids are no longer recommended as first-line therapy for patients with APS without overt lupus, because they are associated with significant foetal and maternal morbidity. Based on data from recent trials, heparin plus low-dose aspirin appears to be the regimen of choice for patients with APS who have a history of thrombosis or pregnancy losses with aspirin alone. Aspirin is safe in pregnancy. Subcutaneous heparin does not cross the placenta and therefore has no adverse effects on the foetus. For the mother, however, potential side effects of heparin treatment include bleeding, thrombocytopenia and osteoporosis. Warfarin must be avoided during the first trimester but may have a role to play subsequently in certain subsets of patients. Some studies have demonstrated that combined therapy with prednisone and aspirin, or with heparin and aspirin, may improve the outcome in women with autoimmune disorders who are undergoing in-vitro fertilization.

Copyright © 1999 S. Karger AG, Basel

Recurrent pregnancy loss (RPL), defined as three or more consecutive spontaneous abortions, affects approximately 1–2% of women of reproductive age. An underlying cause is found in 50% of couples. Alongside

KARGER

Fax + 41 61 306 12 34
E-Mail karger@karger.ch
www.karger.com

© 1999 S. Karger AG, Basel
0301–0147/99/0297–0112$17.50/0

Accessible online at:
www.karger.com/journals/hae

Dr. Bertrand Wechsler
Department of Internal Medicine
Groupe Hospitalier Pitié-Salpêtrière
47-83, Boulevard de l'Hôpital
F–75013 Paris (France)

genetic, anatomic, microbiological and endocrine abnormalities, the antiphospholipid syndrome (APS) is now increasingly recognized as being an important cause.

In 1980, Soulier and Boffa [1] described an association between RPL, thromboembolism and lupus anticoagulant. APS was initially thought to be a haematological form of lupus, but since the studies of Harris and colleagues [2], it has been distinguished from other overt autoimmune disorders such as systemic lupus erythematosus, to which it can be associated.

A prospective study found antiphospholipid antibodies (aPL) to be present in about 15% of cases of recurrent miscarriage [3]. In an unselected population of pregnant women, aPL were found in 2–4% of cases (<1% for lupus anticoagulant) and their positivity was not a good predictor of pregnancy outcome (miscarriage, prematurity, hypotrophy etc.). Consequently, it was considered unwise to search systematically for aPL in unselected pregnancies [4]. Among women with only one miscarriage, there was no significant difference in the prevalence of positive aPL compared with a control population, because of the frequent occurrence of early miscarriage in the general population [5]. On the other hand, the presence of aPL became significant when women with two or more consecutive miscarriages were studied [6].

It is important to note that, in recent prospective studies, women with RPL and aPL who refused to participate and remained untreated had successful pregnancies in less than 10% of cases [7, 8].

In order to clarify the exact relationship between APS and pregnancy loss, Branch and Silver [9] have recently proposed a new nomenclature of pregnancy loss. The approach is to classify pregnancy loss in terms of development periods of gestation: (1) the pre-embryonic period lasts from conception through to 5 weeks from the first day of the last menstrual period; (2) the embryonic period lasts from week 5 through to week 9 of gestation; and (3) the foetal period begins at week 10 of gestation, or 70 days from conception, and extends throughout pregnancy until delivery.

Table 1. Modified obstetric criteria for APS

- One or more otherwise unexplained foetal deaths at or after 10 weeks of gestation, with normal foetal morphology documented by ultrasound or direct examination of the foetus.
- Loss of one or more morphologically normal neonates due to complications of prematurity after delivery for severe pre-eclampsia or evidence of severe placental insufficiency.
- Three or more consecutive pre-embryonic or embryonic losses, with anatomic, genetic and hormonal causes of pregnancy loss excluded.

In the general population, 87% of pregnancy losses occur in the pre-embryonic or embryonic periods. In contrast, in aPL-positive women, the majority of pregnancy losses are foetal deaths. As a result, the obstetric criteria for APS, initially defined as at least two foetal losses [2], have been recently modified (table 1) [9].

The pathogenesis is uncertain, but histologic examination of placentae has suggested that the causal mechanism for pregnancy loss is thrombosis of the utero-placental vasculature [10]. More recent studies have suggested that aPL directly impair trophoblast function, leading to defective implantation and invasion of the uterine decidua. In experimental studies, passive and active induction of anticardiolipin antibodies (aCL) in pregnant mice resulted in a lower fecundity rate, an increased resorption index of embryos, a lower number of embryos per pregnancy and lower weights of embryos and placentae than in control mice [11]. The same group of workers demonstrated that, among diverse therapies, prevention of foetal resorption in mice was achieved with aspirin and with low-molecular-weight heparin (LMWH) [12].

In-vitro studies suggest an increase in thromboxane synthesis [13] and, more recently, a decrease in the distribution of annexin V, a natural placental anticoagulant protein [14] may be responsible.

Therapy

Because APS was initially overdiagnosed as lupus, steroids were thought to be an important part of the therapy.

As early as 1983, Lubbe et al. [15] reported the efficacy of combined therapy with prednisone (40–60 mg/day) and aspirin (75 mg/day) in six women, four of whom had lupus. The five multigravidas had never had a live birth and had had 14 intrauterine deaths. With therapy, five patients completed their pregnancies successfully. One intrauterine death occurred at 16 weeks.

Since then, studies using a variety of treatments, including steroids, aspirin, heparin and immunoglobulin, have been reported. Silveira et al. [16] obtained an overall rate of 100% for live births in women treated with aspirin (81 mg/day) plus prednisone (starting dose 40 mg/day, tapered by 10 mg every 4 weeks to a maintenance dose of 5 mg/day). Four babies were born prematurely. One case of pre-eclampsia, one case of diabetes mellitus and one case of deep venous thrombosis were observed in the mothers. In contrast, in 1989, Lockshin et al. [17] reported worsening of prognosis with prednisone.

Progressively, the role of thrombosis in the pathogenesis has emerged, and antithrombotic therapy has become the leading therapy.

As early as 1990, Rosove et al. [18] reported the beneficial use of heparin alone. They obtained live births in 14 out of 15 instances in 14 women who had a history of 28 miscarriages out of 29 pregnancies. Heparin was administered subcutaneously every 12 h, at a dose adjusted to obtain a mid-interval clotting time of 1.5–2.0 times the control value. The mean total daily dose was 24,700 ± 7,400 IU. These results were recently confirmed by Ruffatti et al. [19], using 5,000 IU of calcium heparin, self-administered by the patients three times a day. They obtained a live-birth rate of 100% in 51 women with a history of 119 miscarriages out of 132 pregnancies. Intravenous immunoglobulins had to be added in two cases.

In 1993, Balasch et al. [20] reported the outcome of treatment with low-dose aspirin alone in 18 women with APS who had a history of 46 miscarriages out of 49 pregnancies. Aspirin (100 mg/day) was started 1 month before attempting conception and continued throughout the pregnancy. Live births were achieved in 19 out of 21 pregnancies. In six pregnancies, prednisone had to be added because of autoimmune-related thrombocytopenia.

A number of trials have been conducted to assess the relative efficiency of the different treatments. In 1992, Cowchock et al. [21] conducted a multicentre randomized trial including 20 patients, comparing aspirin (80 mg/day) plus heparin (administered every 12 h; mean daily dose, 17,000 IU) with aspirin plus prednisone (40 mg/day). The rate of live births was similar in the two treatment groups (75%), but morbidity, mainly preterm delivery with premature rupture of the membranes and pre-eclampsia, was more frequent in the prednisone group. In 1993, Silver et al. [22] randomized patients to receive either prednisone (20 mg/day) plus aspirin (81 mg/day) or aspirin alone. All 34 pregnancies ended in live births, but prednisone therapy was associated with more preterm deliveries (8/12 vs. 3/22). In five of the eight cases, the cause was premature membrane rupture or abruptio placentae.

A significantly lower mean birth weight was also observed in the prednisone group (2,800 vs. 3,350 g).

Moreover, Laskin et al. [23] randomly assigned, in a heterogeneous population, women with at least two foetal losses and one autoantibody (antinuclear, anti-DNA, antilymphocyte, aCL) to receive either prednisone (0.5–0.8 mg/kg/day) and aspirin (100 mg/day) or placebo for the duration of their pregnancy. No significant difference was observed between the two groups for live births (65 and 56% in the treated and placebo groups, respectively), but side effects, especially hypertension and diabetes mellitus, were significantly higher in the treated group (15 vs. 5%).

Since then, for treatment of APS without overt lupus, steroids have fallen into disfavour, because of the significant foetal and maternal morbidity associated with their use.

More recently, two independent trials have shown clearly the benefit of adding heparin to low-dose aspirin in the treatment of aPL-associated RPL [24, 25]. Kutteh [24] conducted a prospective randomized trial of aspirin (81 mg/day) with or without heparin. Heparin dosages were adjusted to maintain 1.2–1.5 times the baseline partial thromboplastin time (PTT). In women treated with heparin plus low-dose aspirin, the live-birth rate was 80%, compared with 44% in women treated with low-dose aspirin alone. Rai et al. [25] conducted a randomized controlled trial of aspirin (75 mg/day) alone versus aspirin plus unfractionated heparin (UFH; 5,000 IU subcutaneously every 12 h). Out of 45 pregnancies in each group, the rate of live births with low-dose aspirin plus heparin was 71% (32 live births), compared with 42% among women treated with low-dose aspirin alone (19 live births, $p = 0.01$).

In practice, in APS, heparin plus low-dose aspirin appears to be the regimen of choice in patients with a history of thrombosis (arterial or venous), a history of pregnancy losses with aspirin alone, or in 'last-chance patients'. In addition to its anticoagulant effect, heparin may act by directly binding aPL in vivo, thereby decreasing their deleterious effects in women with RPL [26]. In other cases, several authors think it might be possible to try aspirin alone initially, in order to simplify therapy. Whatever choice is made, the treatment must be started as soon as the pregnancy test is positive.

Side Effects of Antithrombotic Therapy [27]

Aspirin

Aspirin readily crosses the placenta, but it is known from large studies that aspirin at a low dose (<100 mg/day) is safe in pregnancy [28]. There were no differences between placebo and treated groups in the incidence of excessive blood loss, postpartum haemorrhage, change in haematocrit or the need for transfusions, and no bleeding complications associated with the use of epidural anaesthesia. The incidence of abruptio placentae was superior in the aspirin group but similar to that found in the general population. Similarly, among the neonates, there were no differences in the incidence of cephalohaematoma, cerebral haemorrhage, petechiae, purpura, excessive bleeding at the time of circumcision, any bleeding disorder or the need for transfusion. With a small dosage, there is no risk of premature closure of the arterial canal.

UFH and LMWH

Various dosages of heparin have been used. Hunt et al. [29] proposed to start LMWH (dalteparin) at 5,000 IU (through anti-factor Xa activity levels 0.15 to 0.2 IU/ml). In most of the patients, the dose had to be

Table 2. Dosage schedules and side effects of heparin therapy

Author	Year	Dosage	Aspirin mg/day	Number of women	Thrombo-cytopenia	Fracture	Throm-bosis
Rosove et al. [18]	1990	UFH 10,000 × 2 IU PTT × 2 IU	no	15	0	0	0
Cowchock et al. [21]	1992	UFH 10,000 × 2 IU PTT: high-range normal value	80	12	0	0	1
Kutteh [24]	1996	UFH 5,000 × 2 IU PTT: 1.2–1.5	80	25	0	0	0
Dulitzki et al. [30]	1996	enoxaparin 40 mg, 20 mg (3 patients) 40 mg twice daily (2 high-risk patients)	no	41	0	0	1[a]
Ruffati et al. [19]	1997	UFH 5,000 × 3 IU PTT ≤2	75	53	0	0	0
Hunt et al. [29]	1997	dalteparin 5,000 IU	75	32	0	1[b]	0
Nelson-Piercy et al. [32]	1997	enoxaparin (20 mg) 40 mg × 2 IU (high risk)	75	61	0	0	1[a]
Rai et al. [25]	1997	SCH 5,000 12 hourly	75	45	0	0	0
Backos et al. [31]	1999	enoxaparin 20 mg UFH 5,000 × 2 IU	75 75	150	0	0	0

[a] 20 mg enoxaparin.
[b] Two months postpartum; no other risk factor.
SCH = subcutaneous calcium heparin; PTT: baseline partial thromboplastin time.

increased during the second, and sometimes the third, trimester. Because of the efficacy of the treatment and the risk of osteoporosis, LMWH has been limited to a maximum of 5,000 IU twice daily.

Subcutaneous heparin does not cross the placenta and therefore has no adverse effects on the foetus.

LMWH may offer advantages over standard UFHs: (1) the bioavailability (85–90%) and the longer half-life (3–18 h) allow for once-daily administration; (2) the ratio anti-Xa (antithrombotic)/anti-IIa (anticoagulant) is increased; (3) the release of platelet factor 4 is less important, reducing the risk of late-onset immune thrombocytopenia; (4) the risk of osteoporosis seems diminished (although this was not confirmed in ref. 30); and (5) there is no strict requirement for LMWH discontinuation during surgical procedures [30].

Thrombocytopenia is a potentially dangerous side effect for the mother. It can occur early, or later as an immune-mediated form, which is more serious and associated with paradoxical thrombosis. These complications have to be differentiated from thrombocytopenia commonly seen in APS. Happily, no such complications were documented among nine series of women, totalling 434 cases, receiving UFH and LMWH treatment, compiled from the literature (table 2).

The risk of heparin-induced osteoporosis may be as high as 2%, most frequently subclinical and equivalent to 2 years of postmenopausal bone loss. Nevertheless, the mean decrease in the bone mineral density at the lumbar spine is less than the estimated bone loss as a result of breastfeeding for 6 months [31]. Clinical fractures are seldom observed, and only one is reported in the 434 cumulative cases from the literature (table 2). Bone density improves once heparin therapy is discontinued postpartum. In the series from Nelson-Piercy et al. [32], among 26 women studied with dual-photon X-ray absorptiometry scan, only one with a bone density that was two SDs below the mean had failed to regain bone density when rescanned 15 months later.

Experimental data on rats suggest that heparin-induced osteoporosis is not rapidly reversible because heparin is sequestered in bone for extended periods [33]. It is wise to supplement pregnant patients with calcium (total intake of 1.5 g/day of calcium carbonate) and vitamin D.

Excessive local bruising is rare. To reduce local haematoma formation, it is useful to rotate the injection site and to apply ice to the injection site for several minutes [24].

In view of the high risk of thromboembolism during the immediate postpartum period [34], it is illogical to withhold heparin because of unfounded fears concerning bleeding at the time of delivery, unless the coagulation screen is abnormal. In a cohort of 130 women, 32 out of 94 thrombotic events (34%) occurred during pregnancy and the postpartum period, three of them with 10,000 IU/day of heparin [35]. Lima et al. have reported seven thrombotic events (five venous and two arterial) in 47 women, three of which were observed in the postpartum period as patients were treated with low-dose heparin or aspirin alone [36].

Heparin in low prophylactic doses does not interfere with activation of the normal haemostatic mechanism at the site of injury. If the clotting screen is normal, there is no increased risk of epidural haematoma with epidural/spinal block. In controlled studies, at least 10,000 patients have been given prophylactic doses of LMWH in conjunction with epidural/spinal anaesthesia, without complications. Nevertheless, the catheter has to be inserted at a time greater than 6 h from the previous LMWH injection, or, if appropriate, the next heparin injection can be delayed until after the epidural has been sited [31]. In low-risk pregnancies, the dose of LMWH is omitted immediately before delivery and then treatment is restarted the following day.

Warfarin

Warfarin crosses the placenta, is teratogenic (6–9 GW) and must be avoided during the first trimester. The risk in the second and third trimester is far less clear. The single undisputed indication for warfarin use in pregnancy is for thromboprophylaxis in women with metal prosthetic heart valves. Recently, Hunt et al. [37] described two pregnant women with APS and previous cerebral arterial thrombotic events who relapsed with LMWH. The authors proposed that for women entering pregnancy with high-titre aPL and previous arterial thrombotic events, an elective switch to warfarin, maintaining an international normalized ratio (INR) of 2.5, should be considered at 14 weeks' gestation. Warfarin is continued until 2 weeks before delivery and then switched to intravenous UFH, maintaining an APTT ratio of 2.0–2.5.

Breast-Feeding

Postpartum, neither warfarin nor heparin are excreted in breast milk, and breast-feeding is not contraindicated with their use, this can not be extended for any other coumarin derivative oral coagulants.

Unsolved Problems

Do aPL Have a Pathogenic Role in Infertility?

It has been demonstrated that certain phospholipids are exposed on the endothelial surface and may alter implantation during in-vitro fertilization (IVF). Kaider et al. [38] found a significant difference ($p = 0.01$) in the prevalence of serum aPL in women who failed to conceive after IVF when compared with those who succeeded. However, Birdsall et al. [39], in a similar study, only found a correlation with intrauterine growth retardation.

Treating IVF patients with aspirin, heparin and prednisone remains controversial. Kutteh et al. [40] reported a higher implantation rate in the group of women treated with heparin and aspirin (25 vs. 19.4%) but no statistically significant differences were detected in implantation, pregnancy and ongoing pregnancy rates between those who received standard therapy and those treated with heparin and aspirin. In contrast, Sher et al. [41] reported that treatment with aspirin and heparin was associated with a significant beneficial effect (rate of ongoing pregnancy: 49 vs. 16%, respectively). Similarly, in a retrospective study by Hasegawa et al. [42], treatment with aspirin (81 mg/day) and prednisone (10 mg/day) improved the implantation rate in women with antinuclear antibodies, with or without aPL, who were undergoing IVF.

Is There a Role for Antithrombotic Therapy in Other Conditions?

Immunomodulation has been attempted in women negative for aPL but positive for antithyroid antibodies (antimicrosomal and/or antithyroglobulin) after assisted conception. In a recent study, only 27% of women in the group treated with heparin and aspirin achieved live births, compared with 51% in the group receiving concomitant treatment with intravenous immunoglobin G therapy [43].

Women with Obstetric Features of APS who Have Negative Test Results for Lupus Anticoagulant and Anticardiolipin Antibodies

Silver et al. [44] showed that some women with APS-like syndrome had serum immunoglobulin G pathogenic for murine pregnancy. Randomized trials are needed to determine whether treatments for APS improve pregnancy outcome in such women. Recently, Kupperminc et al. [45], comparing women with normal pregnancies with women without a history of thromboembolism but with severe pre-eclampsia, abruptio placentae, foetal growth retardation and stillbirth, demonstrated that in addition to coagulation inhibitor deficiencies (protein C, protein S, antithrombin III) and aCL (13 vs. 1%), these women also had an increased incidence of mutations predisposing them to thrombosis: mutation at nucleotide 506 in the factor V gene (20 vs. 6%); homozygosis for the C677T mutation in the gene encoding methylene tetrahydrofolate reductase (10 vs. 3%) and mutation G20210A in the prothrombin gene (10 vs. 3%). Similarly, Ridker et al. [46] showed an increased prevalence of factor V Leiden in women with severe pregnancy losses. It is too early to know if antithrombotic therapy will be of any help in such high-risk women.

References

1 Soulier JP, Boffa C: Avortements à répétition, thromboses et anticoagulant circulant anti-thromboplastine. Presse Med 1980;9:859–864.

2 Harris EN, Baguley E, Asherson RA, Hughes GRU: Clinical and serological features of the 'antiphospholipid syndrome'. Br J Rheumatol 1987;26 (suppl 2):19.

3 Clifford K, Rai R, Watson H, Regan L: An informative protocol for the investigation of recurrent miscarriage: Preliminary experience of 500 consecutive cases. Hum Reprod 1994;9:1328–1332.

4 Harris EN, Spinnato JA: Should anticardiolipin tests be performed in otherwise healthy pregnant women? Am J Obstet Gynecol 1991;165: 1272–1277.

5 Infante-Rivard C, David M, Gauthier R, Rivard GE: Lupus anticoagulant, anticardiolipin antibodies, and fetal loss. A case control study. N Engl J Med 1991;325:1063–1066.

6 Kutteh WH, Lyda EC, Abraham SM, Wacholtz MC: Association of anticardiolipin antibodies and pregnancy loss in women with systemic lupus erythematosus. Fertil Steril 1993;60:449–455.

7 Hasegawa I, Takakuwa K, Goto S, Yamada K, Sekizuka N, Kanazawa K, Tanaka K: Effectiveness of prednisone/aspirin therapy for recurrent aborters with antiphospholipid antibody. Hum Reprod 1992;7:203–207.

8 Rai R, Clifford K, Cohen H, Regan L: High prospective fetal loss rate in untreated pregnancies of women with recurrent miscarriage and antiphospholipid antibodies. Hum Reprod 1995;10:3301–3304.

9 Branch DW, Silver RM: Criteria for antiphospholipid syndrome: Early pregnancy loss, fetal loss, or recurrent pregnancy loss? Lupus 1996;5: 409–413.

10 De Wolf F, Carreras LO, Moerman P, Vermylen J, Van Assche A, Renaer M: Decidual vasculopathy and extensive placental infarction in a patient with repeated thromboembolic accidents, recurrent fetal loss, and a lupus anticoagulant. Am J Obstet Gynecol 1982;142:829–834.

11 Shoenfeld Y, Sherer Y, Blank M: Antiphospholipid syndrome in pregnancy – animal models and clinical implications. Scand J Rheumatol 1998;27:S33–S36.

12 Inbar O, Blank M, Faden D, Tincani A, Lorber M, Shoenfeld Y: Prevention of fetal loss in experimental antiphospholipid syndrome by low-molecular-weight heparin. Am J Obstet Gynecol 1993;169:423–426.

13 Peaceman AM, Rehnberg KA: The effect of aspirin and indomethacin on prostacyclin and thromboxane production by placental tissue incubated with immunoglobulin G fractions from patients with lupus anticoagulant. Am J Obstet Gynecol 1995;173:1391–1396.

14 Rand JH, Wu XX, Anree HA, Lockwood CJ, Guller S, Scher J, Harpel PC: Pregnancy loss in the antiphospholipid-antibody syndrome – a possible thrombogenic mechanism. N Engl J Med 1997;337:154–160.

15 Lubbe WF, Butler WS, Palmer SJ, Liggins GL: Fetal survival after prednisone suppression of maternal lupus anticoagulant. Lancet 1983;1: 1361–1363.

16 Silveira LH, Hubble CL, Jara LJ, Saway S, Martinez-Osuna P, Seleznick MJ, Angel J, O'Brien W, Espinoza LR: Prevention of anticardiolipin antibody-related pregnancy losses with prednisone and aspirin. Am J Med 1992;93:403–411.

17 Lockshin MD, Druzin ML, Qamar T: Prednisone does not prevent recurrent fetal death in women with antiphospholipid antibody. Am J Obstet Gynecol 1989;160:439–443.

18 Rosove MH, Tabsh K, Wasserstrum N, Howard P, Hahn BH, Kalunian KC: Heparin therapy for pregnant women with lupus anticoagulant or anticardiolipin antibodies. Obstet Gynecol 1990;75:630–634.

19 Ruffatti A, Orsini A, Di Lenardo L, Nardelli GB, Patrassi GM, Truscia D, Brigato G, Grella P, Todesco S: A prospective study of fifty-three consecutive calcium heparin-treated pregnancies in patients with antiphospholipid antibody related fetal loss. Clin Exp Rheumatol 1997;15: 499–505.

20 Balasch J, Carmona F, Lopez-Soto A, Font J, Creus M, Fabregues F, Ingelmo M, Vanrell JA: Low-dose aspirin for prevention of pregnancy losses in women with primary antiphospholipid syndrome. Hum Reprod 1993;8:2234–2239.

21 Cowchock FS, Reece EA, Balaban D, Branch DW, Plouffe L: Repeated fetal losses associated with antiphospholipid antibodies: A collaborative randomized trial comparing prednisone with low-dose heparin treatment. Am J Obstet Gynecol 1992; 166:1318–323.

22 Silver RK, MacGregor SN, Sholl JS, Hobart J, Neerhof M, Ragin A: Comparative trial of prednisone plus aspirin versus aspirin alone in the treatment of anticardiolipin antibody-positive obstetric patients. Am J Obstet Gynecol 1993;169: 1411–1417.

23 Laskin CA, Bombardier C, Hannah ME, Mandel FP, Ritchie JW, Farewell V, Farine D, Spitzer K, Fielding L, Solonika CA, Yeung M: Prednisone and aspirin in women with autoantibodies and unexplained recurrent fetal loss. N Engl J Med 1997; 337:148–153.

24 Kutteh WH: Antiphospholipid antibody-associated recurrent pregnancy loss: Treatment with heparin and low-dose aspirin to low-dose aspirin alone. Am J Obstet Gynecol 1996; 174:1584–1589.

25 Rai R, Cohen H, Dave M, Regan L: Randomized controlled trial of aspirin and aspirin plus heparin in pregnant women with recurrent miscarriage associated with phospholipid antibodies (or antiphospholipid antibodies). BMJ 1997;314:253–257.

26 Ermel LD, Marshburn PB, Kutteh WH: Interaction of heparin with antiphospholipid antibodies from sera of women with recurrent pregnancy loss. Am J Reprod Immunol 1995; 33:14–20.
27 Nelson-Piercy C: Prevention of thromboembolism in pregnancy. Scand J Rheumatol 1998;27:92–96.
28 Sibai BM, Caritis SN, Thom E, Klebanoff M, McNellis D, Rocco L, Paul RH, Romero R, Witter F, Rosen M for the National Institute of Child Health and Humban Development Network of Maternal-Fetal Medicine Units: Prevention of preeclampsia with low-dose aspirin in healthy, nulliparous pregnant women. N Engl J Med 1993;329:1213–1218.
29 Hunt BJ, Doughty HA, Majumdar G, Copplestone A, Kerslake S, Buchanan N, Hughes G, Khamashta M: Thromboprophylaxis with low molecular weight heparin (Fragmin) in high risk pregnancies. Thromb Haemost 1997;77:39–43.
30 Dulitzki M, Pauzner R, Langevitz P, Pras M, Many A, Schif E: Low-molecular-weight heparin during pregnancy and delivery: Preliminary experience with 41 pregnancies. Obstet Gynecol 1996;87:380–383.
31 Backos M, Rai R, Baxter N, Chilcott IT, Cohen H, Regan L: Pregnancy complications in women with recurrent miscarriage associated with antiphospholipid antibodies treated with low dose aspirin and heparin. Br J Obstet Gynecol 1999;106:102–107.
32 Nelson-Piercy C, Letsky EA, De Swiet M: Low molecular weight heparin for obstetric thromboprophylaxis: Experience of sixty-nine pregnancies in sixty-one women at risk. Am J Obstet Gynecol 1997;176:1062–1068.
33 Shaughnessy SG, Hirsh J, Bhandari M, Muir JM, Young A, Weitz JI: A histomorphometric evaluation of heparin-induced bone loss after discontinuation of heparin treatment in rats. Blood 1999;93:1231–1236.
34 Le Thi Huong D, Weschler B, Edelman P, Fournie A, Le Tallec Y, Piette JC, Godeu: Postpartum cerebral infarction associated with aspirin withdrawal in the antiphospholipid antibody syndrome. J Rheumatol 1993;30:1229–1232.
35 Silver RM, Draper ML, Scott JR, Lyon JL, Reading J, Branch DW: Clinical consequences of antiphospholipid antibodies: A historic cohort study. Obstet Gynecol 1994;83:372–377.
36 Lima F, Khamashta MA, Buchanan NMM, Kerslake S, Hunt BJ, Hughes GR: A study of sixty pregnancies in the patients with the antiphospholipid syndrome. Clin Exp Rheumatol 1996;14:131–136.
37 Hunt BJ, Khamashta M, Lakasing L, Williams FM, Nelson Piercy C, Bewley S, Hughes GR: Thromboprophylaxis in antiphospholipid syndrome pregnancies with previous cerebral arterial thrombotic events: Is warfarin preferable? Thromb Haemost 1998;79:1060–1061.
38 Kaider BD, Price DE, Roussev RG, Coulam CB: Antiphospholipid antibody prevalence in patients with IVF failure. Am J Reprod Immunol 1996;35:388–393.
39 Birdsall MA, Lockwood GM, Ledger WL, Johnson PM, Chamley LW: Antiphospholipid antibodies in women having in-vitro fertilization. Hum Reprod 1996;11:1185–1189.
40 Kutteh WH, Yetman DL, Chantilis SJ, Crain J: Effect of antiphospholipid antibodies in women undergoing in-vitro fertilization. Hum Reprod 1997;12:1171–1175.
41 Sher G, Feinman M, Zouves C, Kuttner G, Maassarani G, Salem R, Matzner W, Ching W, Chong P: High fecundity rates following in-vitro fertilization and embryo transfer in antiphospholipid antibody seropositive women treated with heparin and aspirin. Hum Reprod 1994; 9:2278–2283.
42 Hasegawa I, Yamanoto Y, Murakawa H, Suzuki M, Kurabayaski T, Takakuwa K, Tunaka K: Prednisolone plus low-dose aspirin improves the implantation rate in women with autoimmune conditions who are undergoing in-vitro fertilization. Fertil Steril 1998;70:1044–1048.
43 Sher G, Maassarani G, Zouves C, Feinman M, Sohn S, Matzner W, Chong P, Ching W: The use of combined heparin/aspirin and immunoglobin G therapy in the treatment of in-vitro fertilization patients with antithyroid antibodies. Am J Reprod Immunol 1998;39:223–225.
44 Silver RM, Pierangeli SS, Edwin SS, Umar F, Harris EN, Scott JR, Branch DW: Pathogenic antibodies in women with obstetric features of antiphospholipid syndrome who have negative test results for lupus anticoagulant and anticardiolipin antibodies. Am J Obstet Gynecol 1997;176:628–633.
45 Kupferminc MJ, Eldor A, Steinman N, Many A, Bar-Am A, Jaffa A, Fait G, Lessing JB: Increased frequency of genetic thrombophilia in women with complications of pregnancy. N Engl J Med 1999;340:9–13.
46 Ridker PM, Miletich JP, Buring JE, Ariyo AA, Price DT, Manson JE, Hill JA: Factor V Leiden mutation as a risk factor for recurrent pregnancy loss. Ann Intern Med 1998; 128:1000–1003.

Hæmostasis

Haemostasis 1999;29(suppl 1):121–127

Risk Factors for Thrombosis and Bleedings Prevention of Arterial and Venous Thrombosis Treatment of VTE and Adverse Reactions

1

Hormone Replacement Therapy with 17β-Oestradiol and Risk of Venous Thromboembolism (VTE) – A Population-Based Case-Control Study

E. Høibraaten, M. Abdelnoor, P. M. Sandset

Haematological Research Laboratory, Ullevaal University Hospital, Oslo, Norway

The aim of this population-based case-control study was to evaluate the effect of hormone replacement therapy (HRT) containing natural oestrogens, i.e., 17β-oestradiol, on the risk of venous thromboembolism (VTE). Cases were consecutive females aged 44–70 years discharged from Ullevaal University Hospital with the diagnosis of deep vein thrombosis or pulmonary embolism during 1990–1996. Fifty-one women with cancer-associated thrombosis were excluded from the study. Controls were randomly collected from the same source population and matched by age. The material comprised 176 cases and 352 controls, i.e. two controls for each case. Only formulations containing 17β-oestradiol were used. The frequency of HRT use was 28% (50/176) in cases and 26% (93/352) in controls. The estimated matched crude odds ratio with 95% confidence interval was 1.13 (0.71–1.78), which indicates no significant association of overall use of HRT and VTE. The estimated adjusted odds ratio was 1.22 (0.76–1.94) performing multi-confounded adjustment using the conditional logistic model and adjusting for hypertension, coronary heart disease, diabetes mellitus, smoking habit, BMI and the presence of previous VTE. Stratification for time of exposure indicated an increased risk of VTE, during the first year of use, with a crude odds ratio of 3.54 (1.54–8.2). This effect was reduced by extended use, to a crude odds ratio of 0.66 (0.39–1.10) after the first year of use. This is the first case-control study on the effect of HRT containing only 17β-oestradiol on the risk of VTE. We found no overall association. On subgroup analysis, there was a suggestion that there was a limited increased risk of VTE during the first year of use, but this effect was modified by time of exposure and not found after the first year of use.

2

Mutation Screening in Hungarian Subjects with Low Protein C Activity

M. Dávid H. Losonczy, Á. Nagy, G. Kutscher, M. Meyer

1st Department of Internal Medicine, Medical University of Pécs, Hungary, and Fachhochschule Jena, FB Medizintechnik, Jena, Germany

Hereditary protein C deficiency is responsible for about 2–9% of inherited thrombophilias. Genomic analysis and detailed blood coagulation examinations

KARGER

Fax + 41 61 306 12 34
E-Mail karger@karger.ch
www.karger.com

© 1999 S. Karger AG, Basel

0301–0147/99/0297–0121$17.50/0

Accessible online at:
www.karger.com/journals/hae

of 43 members of 35 Hungarian families with repeatedly low protein C anticoagulant activity have been performed. The mean age of the proposites was 35.53 ± 13.12 years; the male to female ratio, 15/20; their mean age at the time of the thromboembolic episode: 25.69 ± 9.82 years. Twenty-seven (77%) had a positive family history, 13 (37%) had more than one thromboembolic event. Blood coagulation examinations comprised international normalized ratio, fibrinogen, plasminogen, alpha-2-antiplasmin, lupus anticoagulant, activated protein C resistance, protein C, protein S and antihrombin (AT)-III activity and antigen levels. Genetic examinations comprised: genomic DNA isolation with Chelex 100, the presence of FII 20210A allele and FV:Q506 Leiden mutation and for the mutation screening in the protein C gene the combination of polymerase chain reaction (PCR) and denaturing gradient gel electrophoresis (DGGE) or PCR and single-strand conformation polymorphism (SSCP) analysis. The simplified DNA fragments with aberrant migration during DGGE and SSCP analysis were sequenced (ABI Prism 310). Twenty-one members of 15 families (50%) were identified carrying mutations in the protein C gene: one nonsense mutation, one rare frameshift deletion and in 19 patients nine different missense mutations, among them three new mutations (1493 A-G, 35 Asp-Gly; 6231 G-A, 173 Gly-Glu; 8476 C-T, 254 Thr-Ile). The PROC gene mutation was combined with FV:Q506 in five families, type I AT-III deficiency in one family and with type I protein S deficiency in two families. In 19 families no mutations could be identified in their protein C gene: 84% of them had type II deficiency, 11 families (60%) had only a borderline decrease in their protein C activity. The presence of FV:Q506 mutation could be diagnosed in nine families from this group (homozygous in three cases and heterozygous in six cases). In spite of the repeatedly low protein C activity and antigen levels there were six families (17%) without any genetic or blood coagulation alterations. DGGE and SSCP are efficient and money-saving screening methods in the genetic analysis of hereditary protein C deficiency. Three new mutations and a rare frameshift deletion have been proved. Eighty-two percent of families without mutations in the PROC gene (borderline decrease in the protein C activity) had FV:Q506 (Leiden) mutation. In six families there were no detectable coagulation or genetic disturbances. This is the first report about Hungarian families with hereditary protein C deficiency.

3

Thrombocytopenia and Delivery Method as Risk Factors for Intraventricular Haemorrhage in Very-Low-Weight Infants

D.J. Kahn, D.K. Richardson, SNAP II Study Group 2 and H.H. Billett

Division of Hematology, Albert Einstein College of Medicine, Bronx, N.Y., and Departments of Neonatology and Maternal and Child Health, Harvard Medical School, Boston, Mass., USA

We investigated the significance of thrombocytopenia (TP) and delivery method on the incidence of intraventricular haemorrhage (IVH) in 1,453 very-low-birth weight (VLBW) infants (BW <1,500 g) admitted to six neonatal intensive care units over 21 months. Illness severity was measured by the Score for Neonatal Acute Physiology (SNAP), which assesses neonatal status in a 24-h period. A total of 153 infants (10.5%) had TP ($<100 \times 10^9$/l) on day 1 or 3 of admission. Compared with infants without TP, these infants weighed less at birth, had lower gestational ages, higher SNAPs, and lower Apgar scores. More were small for gestational age and had mothers with hypertension. Among non-TP infants, the incidence of IVH (Grades I–IV) was 22.8%; neonates delivered vaginally had more IVH than those delivered by caesarean section (CS) (34.7 vs. 14.8%, $p < 0.001$). Among TP infants, the incidence of IVH was greater (42.9%) and those delivered vaginally had the highest incidence of IVH (62.5 vs. 35.0% for CS, $p < 0.003$). Results for severe IVH (Grades III–IV) were parallel. Multivariate analysis showed delivery method and extreme TP (platelets $<50 \times 10^9$/l) on day 1 to be independent risk factors for IVH (OR 3.0, 95% CI 2.1–4.2 and OR 9.8, 95% CI 2.6–37.5, respectively). This study demonstrates that TP is not infrequent among VLBW infants and that the risk of IVH in these infants is disproportionately high. The incidence of IVH is higher in VLBW infants delivered vaginally and is further increased when these infants have TP. These findings suggest that CS may be of benefit for VLBW infants, especially those at risk for TP.

4

Heparin in Acute Embolic Stroke Trial (HAEST)

Prize-Winning Poster – Best Clinical Study

Eivind Berge, Michael Abdelnoor, Per Morten Sandset

on behalf of the HAEST Study Group, Ullevaal University Hospital, Oslo, Norway

The Heparin in Acute Embolic Stroke Trial (HAEST) was conducted to test whether low-molecular-weight heparin (LMWH) is effective in preventing early stroke recurrence in patients with atrial fibrillation. This was a randomized, double blind and double-dummy, Norwegian multicentre study of patients with atrial fibrillation and acute ischaemic stroke. Patients were randomized within 30 h to treatment with subcutaneous LMWH (dalteparin 100 IU/kg twice a day) or aspirin (160 mg once daily) for 14 days. The Scandinavian Stroke Scale (SSS) was assessed daily. A CT scan was performed at trial entry, after 7 days, and on clinical deterioration. Functional outcomes [Barthel Index, modified Rankin Scale and International Stroke Trial (IST) scale] were determined after 14 days. The IST scale was repeated at final follow-up after 3 months. The primary endpoint was recurrence, defined by a loss of ≥ 3 points in the SSS. Secondary endpoints were functional outcome, change in SSS-score, and death. A total of 449 patients were included. Mean age was 78.8 years. Overall, 54% of the patients were females, 18% were smokers, 39% had hypertension, 34% coronary heart disease, 18% previous transient ischaemic attacks or stroke, 23% heart failure, 14% diabetes and 5% previous venous thromboembolism. Forty-four percent used aspirin, 37% antihypertensive drugs, 24% were on treatment for coronary heart disease and 30% for heart failure. The premorbid modified Rankin Scale was estimated to be 0 or 1 in 84% of the patients. The mean baseline SSS was 35 (max. score 58). According to the OCSP classification, 16% of the strokes were TACIs, 67% PACIs, 12% LACIs and 5% POCIs. In conclusion this is the first randomized study on the use of LMWH in patients with acute stroke and atrial fibrillation.

5

Anticoagulation with Low-Molecular-Weight Heparin (Dalteparin) in Atrial Fibrillation

H. Bechtold, H. Sawitzki, D. Gunzenhauser, D. Janssen

Internal Department of Hospital, Crailsheim and Pharmacia & Upjohn, Erlangen, Germany

In patients with atrial fibrillation, therapeutic anticoagulation is mandatory before and after cardioversion to abolish thromboembolic risks. Low-molecular-weight heparins (LMWH), which are equivalent to unfractionated heparin in the treatment of deep vein thrombosis, might enormously simplify anticoagulation in this setting – i.e. no laboratory controls, no permanent intravenous infusion and ambulant self-administration is possible. We therefore treated 40 patients (20 female, 20 male; aged 42–86 years) consecutively admitted to our hospital with atrial fibrillation (duration 1 day to over 1 year; no prior anticoagulation) with weight-adjusted subcutaneous dalteparin (2 × 100 IU/kg daily, maximal dose 2 × 10,000 IU/day) instead of unfractionated intravenous heparin. All patients gave their written informed consent. In 13 patients with an atrial fibrillation duration of more than 2 days and in whom cardioversion was planned, a transoesophageal echocardiogram (TEE; multiplane probe) was done by an experienced investigator (H.B.) to rule out left atrial or left atrial appendage thrombi. In two patients a left atrial appendage thrombus was detected. Ten of these 13 patients were started on flecainide: six converted to sinus rhythm after 2–3 days and four converted after flecainide pretreatment and electrical cardioversion. Overall, 18 patients out of 40 converted to sinus rhythm, eight spontaneously without active treatment. In none of these patients did a thromboembolic event occur during an in-hospital follow-up of 2–9 days after cardioversion to sinus rhythm. No serious side effects of dalteparin therapy were noted in any of the 40 patients (duration of dalteparin treatment, 4–29 days; mean, 11.8 days). There was no haemorrhagic complications. In one patient, an increase of 40% of GOT and gamma-GT was noted when phenprocoumon was administered simultaneously). Thirty-one patients received an overlapping therapy with the oral anticoagulant drug phenprocoumon before dalteparin was stopped. The activated partial thromboplastin time increased at the time when phenprocoumon and dalteparin were given together (from 34.1 ± 3.28 s at start of dalteparin up to 48.4 ± 9.3 s, n = 24). In conclusion the combination of anticoagulation with the LMWH dalteparin and ruling out left atrial or left atrial appendage thrombi by means of multiplane TEE might enormously simplify and speed up therapy and management of patients with atrial fibrillation, especially if cardioversion is planned. Larger controlled studies are needed to evaluate this new treatment modality.

6

The Use of Thromboprophylaxis in Laparoscopic Surgery in Denmark

M.S. Rasmussen, T.F. Tvedskov, P. Wille-Jørgensen

Department of Surgical Gastroenterology, Bispebjerg Hospital, University of Copenhagen, Denmark

The incidence of thromboembolic complications after laparoscopic surgery is unknown and studies on thromboprophylaxis (TP) in laparoscopic surgery are lacking. Theoretically, the optimal TP for these patients is low-molecular-weight heparin (LMWH) and graded compression stockings. The aim of this study was to determine the current practice of TP during laparoscopic surgery in Denmark. Postal questionnaires were sent to the 55 surgical departments in Denmark, that are performing laparoscopic surgery. Only 39 departments have replied so far. TP was used after firm written instructions in 92% of the responding departments. Fourteen departments used TP for all patients, and only three departments used TP sporadically. All departments used LMWH as TP, 77% in combination with graded compression stockings. Almost a quarter of the departments had experienced symptomatic thromboembolic complications following laparoscopic surgery. We conclude that the majority of surgical departments in Denmark use TP after firm written instructions in connection with laparoscopic surgery. All departments use LMWH, usually in combination with graded compression stockings.

7

Ten Consecutive Successful Pregnancies in Women with Thrombocytosis due to Myeloproliferative Diseases Receiving Prophylactic Aspirin Therapy

S.I. Allen, W. Zaheer, S. Lichtman, L. Weiselberg

Department of Medicine, North Shore University Hospital, Manhasset, N.Y., USA

Myeloproliferative disorders are being recognized more frequently in young adults. A high risk for spontaneous abortion, especially during the first trimester, has been reported in women with essential thrombocythaemia. Aspirin prophylaxis has been recommended as a therapy. We report our prospective experience with 10 consecutive pregnancies in six patients who were treated with aspirin throughout pregnancy. Pregnant patients with thrombocytosis due to essential thrombocythaemia (four patients) or polycythaemia vera (two patients) were treated with prophylactic aspirin therapy. Serial medical evaluations and complete blood counts were obtained throughout their pregnancies and in the postpartum period. Maternal platelet counts decreased during all 10 pregnancies. There was no significant bleeding, nor thrombotic complications. All patients delivered full-term, normal babies. In conclusion aspirin appears to be a safe and effective prophylactic medication in this clinical setting.

8

Monitoring Heparin Therapy Based on TAT- and D-Dimer Values Does Not Help: Experience with 305 High-Risk Pregnancies

T. Bombeli, P.R. Mueller, J. Fehr

Coagulation Laboratory, Division of Haematology, University of Zurich, Switzerland

The true risk of thrombosis for women with thrombophilia or a history of thrombosis is not known. Consequently, the indication and use of heparin as thromboprophylaxis varies widely. Since coagulation activation markers can indicate an increased risk of thrombosis and are sensitive to heparin therapy, we tested whether thrombin-antithrombin III complexes (TAT) and D-dimers are useful for risk assessment and heparin monitoring. During 6 years, 261 women (305 pregnancies) with hereditary or acquired thrombophilia, a personal or family history of thrombosis, or with thrombosis in the current pregnancy were closely monitored with TAT and D-dimers. As soon as one TAT or D-dimer value was above the cut-off value, thromboprophylaxis was started using either unfractionated heparin (UFH) or low-molecular-weight heparin (LMWH). The subsequent doses were adjusted solely on the basis of TAT and D-dimers values. The data were analysed retrospectively. More than 95% of the patients had had an increased TAT or D-dimer value and were treated with heparin. In 66% of the pregnancies, the mean value of all TAT values of the entire pregnancy was above the cut-off. Increased TAT values were found primarily during the second half of the pregnancy. There were no differences of the TAT or D-dimer values and consequently the heparin doses between the different thrombophilia groups, except for the group with thrombosis in the current pregnancy, which had significantly higher values and heparin doses. The TAT values were suppressed more effectively by LMWH than by UFH. The doses of UFH and LMWH increased continuously with the gestational age (the mean daily dose was 10,800 and 4,100 IU, respectively). There were only two deep venous thromboses out of 8,439 treatment weeks. We conclude that the establishment of anticoagulant therapy with TAT and D-dimers is feasible but does not help. However, it does not help to assess the gestational risk and it seems that too many women are treated unnecessarily. Also, very high doses of heparin may be required by the end of the pregnancy. All in all, there are no major advantages of using activation markers for heparin monitoring that outweigh the high expenses and efforts of the patients.

9

Supratherapeutic Levels of Heparin Anticoagulation Result in Increased Complications

C.J. Della Valle, L.M. Jazrawi, J.D. Zuckerman, P.E. Di Cesare

Department of Orthopedic Surgery, New York University-Hospital for Joint Diseases, New York, N.Y., USA

The purposes of this study were to determine whether bleeding complications associated with the use of intravenous heparin after major orthopaedic operations are as prevalent as has previously been reported and to identify factors predictive of these events so that they can be avoided. Sixty-eight consecutive patients who received 72 courses of intravenous heparin therapy for the treatment of thromboembolic complication after major orthopaedic operations were retrospectively reviewed. Anticoagulation with intravenous heparin was initiated a mean of 4 days postoperatively (range 2–13 days), and 82% of patients received an initial heparin bolus. Major complications were defined as wound related (haematoma, infection or dehiscence), non-operative haemorrhage (i.e. gastrointestinal), recurrent thromboembolism, arterial thrombosis, heparin-induced thrombocytopenia, transfusion of >2 units of blood or a fall in haemoglobin >2 g/dl. Minor complications were defined as thrombocytopenia (platelet count < 100,000/dl or a decrease of >200,000/dl) or other minor bleeding episodes. The bleeding complication rate was 14% (10 of 72). Patients who suffered a bleeding complication during treatment for thromboembolism with intravenous heparin had a mean maximal activated partial thromboplastin time (APTT) that was significantly higher (more than twice recommended levels) when compared with those who did not ($p < 0.05$). Unmatched logistic regression analysis revealed the maximal APTT as the only independent variable predictive of bleeding events (odds ratio 33.4; $p < 0.05$). We conclude that bleeding complications can be minimized and heparin administered safely in the early post-operative period if coagulation parameters are closely monitored and maintained within recommended levels (1.5 to 2.0 times control). Patients with an APTT greater than 90 seconds are at high risk for bleeding complications.

10

A Novel Technique Combining Local Thrombolysis with Thrombectomy for the Treatment of Acute Deep Vein Thrombosis

J. Largiader, B. Gloor, A. Bellaria

Centre for Vascular Diseases, Zurich, Switzerland

We report a procedure developed to restore patency and preserve valve function in acute deep vein thrombosis (DVT) as well as early clinical results. Under general anaesthesia, the thrombosed leg is excluded from the circulation by a tourniquet applied to the upper thigh. Urokinase (2–4 million IU) and heparin (5,000 IU) are infused through a cannula placed in a dorsal foot vein prior to the operation. The lytic agent is allowed to act for 20–30 min. Meanwhile, the femoral vein is opened and pelvic thrombectomy is performed, if necessary. The tourniquet is then removed and the thrombi, now freely floating, are washed out by the enormous flow resulting from reactive hyperaemia. Control venography is performed through the cannula and the procedure repeated if residual thrombi are observed. The patient is then given heparin, phenprocoumon and compression hosiery (Sigvaris® 503). Fifty-six patients (mean age 41 years, 86% with whole leg and/or pelvic DVT, 66% with symptoms of 5 days or less) were treated according to this scheme. Overall 41% experienced wound haematoma requiring drainage and 50% needed blood transfusions. No other adverse events were recorded. A total of 21% underwent additional procedures to secure outflow (pelvic stent or crossover bypass). At follow-up (median interval 34 months) 45 patients (80%) had patent veins and competent valves as judged from duplex examination. The procedure described combines the advantages of local thrombolysis with those of thrombectomy, avoiding many of the complications of either method. The mid-term results are excellent. We therefore continue to use the technique in acute massive DVT, especially in young people with a short history and no known thrombophilia.

11

Treatment of Antiphospholipid Antibody Syndrome with High-Dose Dalteparin

L.A. Valentino, J. Meserow, A. Taylor
Rush University, Chicago, Ill., USA

Antiphospholipid antibody syndrome (APLAS) refers to the association of antiphospholipid antibodies (APLA) with recurrent foetal loss, thrombosis and thrombocytopenia. Obstetric complications include recurrent miscarriages, foetal death, intrauterine growth retardation, preterm delivery, early and/or severe pre-eclampsia, abruptio placentae and utero-placental insufficiency. The pathogenesis of APLAS is thought to be due to APLA-induced platelet hyperaggregability, decreased endothelial prostacyclin synthesis and inhibition of natural anticoagulants. Management of APLAS during pregnancy is controversial but includes anticoagulation. Recent success with low-molecular-weight heparins (LMWHs) in venous thromboembolism has prompted LMWH use in APLAS. We report the successful use of high-dose LMWH to treat APLAS.

Our patient, a 36-year-old woman, presented in the 18th week of her eighth pregnancy. Her first three pregnancies had ended with foetal demise and spontaneous abortion at 13, 20 and 29 weeks' gestation, respectively. Her fourth pregnancy had ended at 23 weeks' gestation despite treatment with steroids, aspirin and fixed-dose unfractionated heparin (UFH). During her fifth and sixth pregnancies, she had been treated with progesterone, steroids, aspirin and UFH, but foetal demise had occurred at 8 and 7 weeks' gestation, respectively. Prior to the seventh pregnancy, the patient had been treated with intravenous immunoglobulin (IVIG), then with aspirin and UFH following conception. Foetal demise had occurred at 8 weeks' gestation. Prior to and following the eighth conception, she was treated with IVIG along with aspirin, progesterone and UFH until the 18th week of gestation. At that time, anti-factor Xa activity was undetectable. The patient was converted to LMWH (dalteparin), at a dose ranging from 5,000 IU twice daily to 10,000 IU three times a day, to maintain anti-factor Xa activities of 0.15–0.20 IU/ml just prior to the next dose and 0.40–0.60 IU/ml 2 h after administration of LMWH. Ecchymoses were present at the injection sites but no serious bleeding complications were noted. A healthy male infant was delivered at 37 weeks' gestation.

12

Heparin/Platelet Factor 4 Antibodies Following Multiple Re-exposure to Unfractionated Heparins

F. Mertzlufft, M. Loebe, A. Koster, H. Kuppe, R. Hetzer
Departments of Anaesthesiology and Intensive Care, University of Homburg-Saar, and Departments of Cardiothoracic Surgery and Anaesthesiology, German Heart Centre, Berlin, Germany

Heparin-induced thrombocytopenia type II (HIT II) is a life-threatening complication of any heparin therapy. This frequently poses a major problem in patients being prepared for cardiac surgery, for which a high prevalence of heparin/platelet factor 4 antibodies (ca. 20%) has been described [1]. The present goal was to analyse the impact of multiple episodes of heparinization with unfractionated heparins (UFHs) on the prevalence of these antibodies. A total of 55 patients scheduled for ventricular mechanical assistance participated. All patients had a history of multiple re-exposure (n = 5) to UFHs. Data were collected before surgery with the platelet factor 4 enzyme-linked immunosorbent assay PF 4 ELISA. In 27 of the patients (nearly 50%), the heparin/platelet factor 4 ELISA gave a positive result (optical density >500); i.e. there was an increase in the antibody activity. This result means that the patients are more likely to get HIT. Adequate management of the cardiac patient with HIT II is crucial to the outcome. Obviously, preoperative management must focus on the marked increase in heparin/platelet factor 4 antibodies associated with the re-exposure to UFHs, which usually occurs. However, further evidence is required to correlate the present results with the clinical symptoms of HIT II. Remarkably, occurrence of such antibodies was markedly increased (80%) in stored samples (>2 years). This might be related to an artefact caused by either stored cryo-samples or a different immunogenicity due to different preparations and/or charges of the heparins.

Reference

1 Bauer TL, Arepally G, Konkle BA, Mestichelli B, Shapiro SS, Cines DB, Poncz M, McNutty S, Amiral J, Hauck WW, Edie RN, Mannion JD: Prevalence of heparin-associated antibodies without thrombosis in patients undergoing cardiopulmonary bypass surgery. Circulation 1997;95:1242–1246.

13

Heparin-Induced Thrombocytopenia (HIT): Interest and Difficulties to Identify the Immunologic Mechanism in Patients Treated for Venous Thromboembolism

L. Eialawy, C. Lecrabier, F. Potevin, J. Conard, M.H. Horellou, L. Gonin-Thibsuh, M.M. Samama

Hématologie Biologique, Hôpital Hôtel-Dieu, Paris, France

In patients treated for venous thromboembolism (VTE), heparin-induced thrombocytopenia (HIT) is very rare but potentially life-threatening. Previous studies have reported heterogeneous populations and many patients had other diseases inducing thrombocytopenia. We have examined 24 consecutive patients treated with heparin for VTE. They were referred for an abrupt fall of platelet count during treatment, without known cancer, sepsis, or concomitant therapy causing thrombocytopenia. There is no gold-standard diagnostic criteria and the diagnosis of HIT is difficult. We have established a score with anamnestic criteria, which allowed us to compare two biological tests: platelet aggregation test (PAT) and an ELISA test (Heparin Platelet Induced Antibodies, HPIA, Stago). The study group consisted of eight men and 16 women with a mean ageof 65 ± 5.6 years (range 27–91 years). Twelve patients received unfractionated heparin, and 12 low-molecular-weight heparin for deep vein thrombosis (n = 16), pulmonary embolism (n = 2) or both (n = 6). Thrombocytopenia appeared within 10.4 ± 8 days (range 1–29 days) with a decrease of over 50% of the initial value of platelet count. Clinical complications occurred in eight patients: extension of venous thrombosis in four, successfully treated with danaparoid, arterial thrombosis in three, leading to death in one patient, and a giant urticaria. Platelet count normalization occurred in 4.5 ± 3.1 days (range 2–10 days) except in four patients, who died despite danaparoid treatment in three of them, suggesting an in-vivo cross reactivity.

Clinical score/ Laboratory tests	Very likely	Likely	Possible	Unlikely
PAT + and HPIA +	10	2	1	0
PAT – and HPIA –	0	0	2	1
PAT + and HPIA –	2	2	4	0
PAT – and HPIA +	0	0	0	0

The sensitivity and negative predictive value of PAT are superior to those of HPIA, which is more specific. Good clinical scoring in combination with both tests will be very helpful in the difficult diagnosis of HIT.

Hæmostasis

Haemostasis 1999;29(suppl 1):128–129

Conclusion

Sylvia Haas[a] Mark Levine[b] Meyer-Michel Samama[c]

[a] Institut für Experimentelle Onkologie und Therapieforschung, Technical University, Munich, Germany, [b] Hamilton Regional Cancer Centre, Hamilton Ont., Canada, [c] Hôpital Hôtel-Dieu, Paris, France

Substantial progress has been achieved in the field of thromboembolism. However, some important questions have remained unanswered, and several of these were chosen by the programme committee for discussion at this symposium.

The risk factors for venous thromboembolism (VTE) are well documented and it is recognized that thrombosis is a multicausal disease – interactions occur between genetic and acquired risk factors. It has become clear that different types of acquired thromobophilia exist. Additionally, in acquired thrombophilia, hyperhomocysteinaemia does not have the same importance as the antiphospholipid syndrome. The current aim of investigators is to discover new mutations to evaluate which patients are at risk of venous thrombosis, or the risk of VTE in an individual patient.

In an attempt to evaluate these risks, a clinical algorithm was proposed, which stratifies patients into low, medium or high risk of deep vein thrombosis (DVT). It is thought that if D-dimer testing is included in the algorithm, the strategy will be improved. This exciting approach, however, requires validation. In addition, although D-dimer has aided diagnosis of VTE, further research is required to determine the optimal D-dimer laboratory test and how best to incorporate this test into the clinical algorithm. The diagnosis of pulmonary embolism (PE) has been improved by the addition of both chest computed tomography (CT) and D-dimer measurements.

The treatment of choice for acute venous thrombosis is rapidly becoming low-molecular-weight heparin (LMWH), and outpatient treatment should be considered for this condition. Contraindications to outpatient treatment, however, include patients at high risk of haemorrhage and those with comorbid diseases that preclude them from being at home.

The question concerning the duration of prophylaxis in patients undergoing major orthopaedic surgery is still under debate. Controversy, however, also exists over the endpoints that should be used in clinical studies in order to assess the long-term benefit of any VTE prophylaxis. For instance, well-designed, double-blind, randomized, placebo-controlled studies have provided evidence that extending LMWH prophylaxis beyond the hospital stay – for up to 4–5 weeks postoperatively – can significantly reduce the rates

KARGER

Fax + 41 61 306 12 34
E-Mail karger@karger.ch
www.karger.com

© 1999 S. Karger AG, Basel

Accessible online at:
www.karger.com/journals/hae

of venographically proven DVT. The clinical importance of these venographically detected asymptomatic thrombi has, however, provoked vigorous and controversial discussion.

The results of a recent study in hip surgery generated discussion in another area of controversy: the question of commencing prophylaxis pre- or post-operatively. The North American Fragmin Trial (NAFT) was the first to demonstrate that preoperative prophylaxis may be superior to post-operative prophylaxis. However, this study failed to detect a significant difference in post-operative DVT between the two groups.

Although oral anticoagulants, aspirin and heparin are well-established drugs for treatment of both venous and arterial thromboembolism, the search for new and safe antithrombotic drugs is ongoing. Numerous antithrombotic agents are still at an early stage of investigation; however, there have been a number of recent advances. For example, low-molecular-weight thrombin inhibitors are currently being tested for use in patients with heparin-induced thrombocytopenia and, so far, results appear to be quite positive.

Regarding prophylaxis of VTE during pregnancy, current evidence is based only on case histories. It has been recognized that previous VTE episodes and/or hereditary or acquired thrombophilia are the major indications for antithrombotic prophylaxis in pregnancy. Debate over initiation of treatment, however, is still ongoing. Most experts recommend prophylaxis to be used throughout the pregnancy, while others consider refraining from prophylaxis until the second or third trimester of pregnancy.

Anticoagulation for pregnant women with mechanical heart valves remains a problematic issue for physicians. No large randomized trials have been carried out and it is unlikely that such a trial will be carried out in the future.

Although for many years oral anticoagulants have not been recommended for treatment of pregnant women, the pendulum is now shifting towards their use for a defined period in pregnant women with venous thromboembolism or mechanical heart valves.

Data from several large-scale studies have shown that LMWH compounds are significantly more efficacious compared with placebo and may be superior to unfractionated heparin in the setting of unstable coronary syndromes. Once again, controversy prevails over the duration of treatment in patients with this disease. The important role heparins and heparan sulphate play, not only in haemostasis but also in other important biological processes, was discussed. The latter may potentially play a role in the ageing process and diabetes.

A possible use for heparins that has not been studied widely is as antineoplastic agents to prevent the spread of cancer. A comprehensive review of the potential impact of malignant cells on haemostasis was presented. Experimental findings favour the use of heparins as antineoplastics in cancer patients but clinical data are limited. The time has come for definitive large-scale clinical trials to be carried out.

Finally, heparin may play an important role in diabetic microangiopathy. However, it is unknown if this activity is related to anticoagulant or non-anticoagulant activities of heparin.

Many interesting and enlightening papers were presented at the symposium. The final presentation, however, was one of special note; Nobel Laureate Louis Ignarro of UCLA gave an elegant and personal presentation detailing the role of nitric oxide in systemic disease.

We hope that you found these proceedings helpful and informative, and we look forward to seeing you next year at the 7th symposium.

Hæmostasis

Author Index

KARGER

Fax + 41 61 306 12 34
E-Mail karger@karger.ch
www.karger.com

© 1999 S. Karger AG, Basel

Accessible online at:
www.karger.com/journals/hae

Subject Index

KARGER
Fax + 41 61 306 12 34
E-Mail karger@karger.ch
www.karger.com

© 1999 S. Karger AG, Basel

Accessible online at:
www.karger.com/journals/hae